MW00745423

Prostate Cancer

Edited by

William K. Oh
Clinical Director
Lank Center for Genitourinary Oncology
Dana-Farber Cancer Institute
Harvard Medical School
Boston, MA, USA

John Logue
Consultant Oncologist
Clinical Oncology Department
Christie Hospital NHS Trust
Manchester, UK

Series Editor
Arthur T. Skarin
Associate Professor of Medicine
Harvard Medical School
Senior Attending Physician
Medical Director, Lowe Center for Thoracic Oncology
Dana-Farber Cancer Institute
Department of Medicine, Brigham and Women's Hospital
Boston, MA, USA

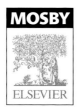

EDINBURGH LONDON NEW YORK OXFORD
PHILADELPHIA ST LOUIS SYDNEY TORONTO 2007

ELSEVIER
MOSBY

© 2003, Elsevier Limited.
© 2007 this compilation, Elsevier Limited. All rights reserved.
First published 2007

ISBN: 978 0 7234 3436 8

British Library Cataloguing in Publication Data
A catalogue record for this book is available from the British Library.

Library of Congress Cataloging in Publication Data
A catalog record for this book is available from the Library of Congress.

Note
Knowledge and best practice in this field are constantly changing. As new research and experience broaden our knowledge, changes in practice, treatment and drug therapy may become necessary or appropriate. Readers are advised to check the most current information provided (i) on procedures featured or (ii) by the manufacturer of each product to be administered, to verify the recommended dose or formula, the method and duration of administration, and contraindications. It is the responsibility of the practitioner, relying on their own experience and knowledge of the patient, to make diagnoses, to determine dosages and the best treatment for each individual patient, and to take all appropriate safety precautions. To the fullest extent of the law, neither the Publisher nor the Editors/Authors assume any liability for any injury and/or damage to persons or property arising out or related to any use of the material contained in this book.

The Publisher

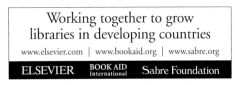

Working together to grow
libraries in developing countries

www.elsevier.com | www.bookaid.org | www.sabre.org

ELSEVIER   BOOK AID International   Sabre Foundation

your source for books,
journals and multimedia
in the health sciences
www.elsevierhealth.com

The
Publisher's
policy is to use
**paper manufactured
from sustainable forests**

Printed in China

Contents

Preface

The increasing incidence and variable natural history of prostate cancer presents a challenge to all professionals involved in its management. The clinical and scientific understanding of this disease is rapidly changing, and with it its management.

This book provides a review of the current state of knowledge in defining the disease process and its optimal management. Prostate cancer remains unique in its ability to remain latent in a proportion of men, making decisions regarding population screening and individual treatment challenging.

A review of its epidemiology and the evolving role of molecular markers in the characterization of malignancies provides insight into defining the behaviour of disease, allowing appropriate treatment to match. A full and detailed review of pathology leads on to a detailed synopsis of current evidence-based therapy. The evolving role of systemic therapy is detailed, and a succinct review outlines potential future drug strategies, examining current investigational drugs and highlighting potential pathways that could be targeted.

A final chapter examines the occurrence and management of systemic and myocutaneous reactions to systemic therapy, which are now being increasingly seen in the clinic as a result of the intensification of therapy and the integration of new biological agents.

The increase in the number of screen-detected prostate cancers in Europe follows the pattern seen in the US; many of the treatment paradigms raised by this change have been addressed in the US and are expounded in this book

John Logue
Consultant Oncologist
Clinical Oncology Department
Christie Hospital NHS Trust,
Manchester, UK

Contributors

Christopher L. Corless, MD, PhD
Professor of Pathology
Oregon Health and Science University
Portland, OR, USA

Joseph P. Eder, MD
Assistant Professor of Medicine, Harvard Medical School
Phase I Group
Medical Oncology Division
Dana-Farber Cancer Institute
Department of Medicine
Brigham and Women's Hospital
Boston, MA, USA

Marc B. Garnick, MD
Clinical Professor
Department of Medicine, Divison of Hematology and Oncology
Harvard Medical School
Beth Israel Deaconess Medical Center
Editor in Chief, *Perspectives on Prostate Disease*,
a publication of Harvard Medical School
Boston, MA, USA

Philip W. Kantoff, MD
Professor of Harvard Medical School
Chief Clinical Research Officer
Chief, Division of Solid Tumor Oncology and Director,
Lank Center for Genitourinary Oncology,
Dana-Farber Cancer Institute,
Boston, MA, USA

Janina A. Longtine, MD
Assistant Professor of Pathology, Harvard Medical School
Clinical Director, Molecular Biology Laboratory
Department of Pathology
Brigham and Women's Hospital
Boston, MA, USA

Mari Nakabayashi, MD, PhD
Research Associate
Lank Center for Genitourinary Oncology
Department of Medical Oncology
Dana-Farber Cancer Institute
Boston, MA, USA

Robert W. Ross, MD
Attending Physician
Lank Center for Genitourinary Oncology
Dana-Farber Cancer Institute
Harvard Medical School
Boston, MA, USA

Tad Wieczorek, MD
Instructor in Pathology, Harvard Medical School
Department of Pathology
Brigham and Women's Hospital
Boston, MA, USA

Acknowledgements

The work of the associate editors of the *Atlas of Diagnostic Oncology* needs to be acknowledged. Dr Maxine Jochelson (currently Director of Oncologic Radiology and Women's Imaging, Cedars-Sinai Medical Center, Los Angeles, CA) and Dr Robert Penny (currently Director of Hematopathology, Community and St Vincent's Hospital of Indianapolis, IN) assisted with the first edition. Their immense help in organizing and evaluating the radiographic and pathology material for the chapters contributed significantly to the success of the *Atlas*. The work of the associate editors of the third edition, Dr Kitt Shaffer, Clinical Director of Radiology at Dana-Farber Cancer Institute and Dr Tad Wieczorek, Clinical Fellow in Pathology at Brigham and Women's Hospital, is also deeply appreciated. Their expertise was invaluable in emphasizing the illustrative and teaching aspects of the third edition. Without their hard work on the *Atlas of Diagnostic Oncology* this Handbook would not have been possible.

Acknowledgement also has to go to the editorial staff at Elsevier Ltd for their assistance in preparing the *Dana-Farber Cancer Institute Handbook Series*.

Introduction

1

Arthur T. Skarin

Worldwide, an estimated 11 million new cases and 7 million cancer deaths occurred in 2002, while nearly 25 million people were living with cancer.[1] Global disparities in cancer incidence, mortality and prevalence relate to genetic susceptibility and ageing, but also to modifiable risk factors such as tobacco abuse, infectious agents, diet (low fruit and vegetable consumption) and physical activity. Other modifiable factors include overweight/obesity, urban air pollution, indoor smoke from household fires, unsafe sex, and contaminated injections in healthcare settings.[2] At least one-third of world cancer deaths are felt to be preventable. The associations of established causes of human cancers have been categorized as chemicals and naturally occurring compounds, medicines and hormones, infectious agents and mixtures.[3]

Due to improvements in healthcare and other factors, there is an increasing ageing population in the US and many other countries in the world. It has been estimated that the proportion of people over age 65 will increase in the US from 12.6% in 2000 to 14.7% in 2015, and 20% in 2030.[4] This compares with 18.1% in Italy (used as a comparison as the oldest country in the world) in 2000, 22.2% in 2015, and 28.1% in 2030. Since the incidence of cancer increases with age, a rising number of cancer cases and deaths is predicted. Screening for cancer is therefore extremely important for early detection and subsequent cure. The annual screening recommendations by the American Cancer Society have been published.[5] To screen for prostate cancer, men over age 50 with a life expectancy of 10 or more years should have annual digital rectal examination and a prostate-specific antigen blood test.

The likelihood of developing cancer during one's lifetime is one in two for males compared with one in three for females, based on 1998–2000 Surveillance, Epidemiology, and End Results data.[6] However, the median age at cancer diagnosis is higher for men at 68 years compared with 65 years for women. The overall 5-year relative survival rate for all patients is 62.7% with considerable variation by cancer site and stage at diagnosis. The variation in cancer statistics in males over recent years in the US is depicted in Figures 1.1 and 1.2. The American Cancer Society estimated that in 2006 the total number of new cases of cancer in men at all sites would be 720,280 with 291,270 deaths (see Figure 1.3).[7] The death rate from all cancers combined has decreased by 1.5% per year since 1993 among men. Indeed, the mortality rate in men has continued to decrease for the three most common sites (lung/bronchus, colon/rectum and prostate). Of interest, since 1999, cancer has surpassed heart disease as the leading cause of death for those under age 85.[7] The reverse exists for those over age 85.

Cancer prevention is extremely important and the progress in information technology has been recently reviewed.[8] Chemoprevention studies have been carried out for several cancers and also recently reviewed.[9] The lifetime risk of developing prostate cancer is 19% in the US. In this setting, risk factors include older age, positive family history of prostate cancer, race, ethnicity and possibly dietary fat.[10] Based upon detailed risk factor assessment worldwide, it is possible that a diet rich in vegetables and low in meat and animal fat may reduce the incidence of prostate cancer.[1]

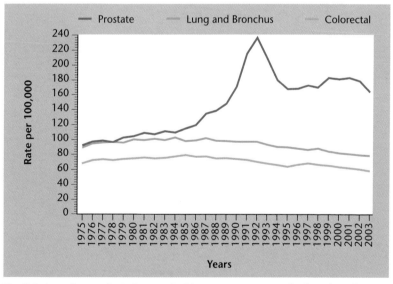

Fig. 1.1 Annual age-adjusted cancer incidence rates among males for selected cancers in the US, 1975–2002. Data from: Surveillance, Epidemiology, and End Results (SEER) program (http://seer.cancer.gov) SEER*Stat Database: Incidence – SEER 9 Regs Public-Use, Nov 2005 Sub (1973–2003), National Cancer Institute, DCCPS, Surveillance Research Program, Cancer Statistics Branch, released April 2006, based on the November 2005 submission.

In 2003, a large chemoprevention trial showed a decrease in the incidence of prostate cancer. This involved the use of finasteride (5 mg), which decreased prostate cancer to an incidence of 18.4% vs. 24.4% in the control arm, for an overall 24.8% reduction over 7 years (p <0.001).[11] Nonetheless, this trial has been controversial because of a higher incidence of higher-grade cancers, and routine finasteride use has not been adapted. More trials are ongoing, and it is expected that progress in chemoprevention will accelerate. This topic has been recently reviewed in detail.[12] Among the goals of these trials are to integrate correlative biomarker expressions into the development of new agents for chemoprevention. The molecular targets summarized in this American Association for Cancer Research Task Force Report included anti-inflammatory/antioxidant agents, epigenetic modulation areas and signal transduction modulation targets. Six characteristics of neoplasms and the associated molecular targets that may be adversely affected by chemoprevention or definitive treatment programmes are noted in Table 1.1.[12]

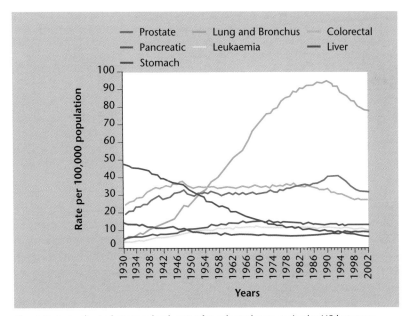

Fig. 1.2 Age-adjusted cancer death rates for selected cancers in the US between 1930 and 2002 for males. Source: US Mortality Public Use Data Tapes, 1960–2002, US Mortality Volumes, 1930–1959, National Center for Health Statistics, Centers for Disease Control and Prevention, 2005. Reproduced with permission from American Cancer Society. Cancer facts and figures 2006. Atlanta, American Cancer Society, Inc.

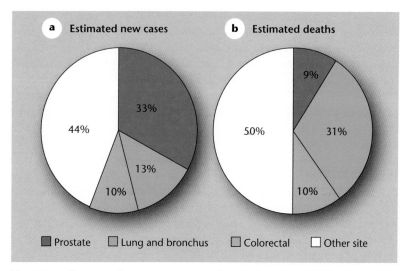

Fig. 1.3 Leading sites of new cancer cases and deaths in males – 2006 estimates. (a) Estimated new cases (b) Estimated deaths. Source: American Cancer Society, Inc., Surveillance Research. Estimates of new cases are based on incidence rates from 1979 to 2002, National Cancer Institute's Surveillance, Epidemiology, and End Results program, nine oldest registries. Estimates of deaths are based on data from US Mortality Public Use Data Tapes, 1969–2003, National Center for Health Statistics, Centers for Disease Control and Prevention, 2006.

The effect of inflammation in the pathogenesis of prostate cancer has been recently reviewed.[13] This appears to be important in the peripheral zone of the prostate where most lesions of intraepithelial neoplasia and invasive adenocarcinoma are observed.

Prostate cancer risk is strongly related to family history. With completion of the Human Genome Project new knowledge has become available about genetic variations that can help to understand the family history as a risk factor for most cancer types. Identification of mutations in genes may identify individuals at high risk for certain cancers (e.g. BRCA1, BRCA2, p53, PTEN and others), allowing for early detection, as well as increased understanding of the aetiological subtypes of cancer and inherited alterations in drug metabolism. This exciting field of molecular epidemiology may thus impact favourably on cancer prognosis.[14] The importance of the above underscores the need for collection and storage of adequate tumour tissue for study.

The new information explosion in molecular biology has led to important discoveries in unique patterns of gene expression characteristic of

Table 1.1 Molecular biomarkers associated with neoplasia characteristics[12]

Evading apoptosis

BCL-2, BAX, caspases, FAS, TNF receptor, DR5, IGF/PI3K/AKI, mTOR, p53, PTEN, *ras*, IL-3, NF-κB

Insensitivity to antigrowth signals

SMADs, pRb, cyclin-dependent kinases, MYC

Limitless replicative potential

hTERT, pRb, p53

Self-sufficiency in cell growth

Epidermal growth factor, platelet-derived growth factor, MAPK, PI3K

Sustained angiogenesis

VEGF, basic fibroblast growth factor, $\alpha_v\beta_3$, thrombospondin-1, hypoxia-inducible factor-1α

Tissue invasion and metastasis

Matrix metalloproteinases, MAPK, E-cadherin

BAX, BCL-2 associated X protein
BCL-2, B cell lymphoma 2
DR5, death receptor 5
FAS, fatty acid synthase
hTERT, human telomerase reverse transcriptase
IGF, insulin-like growth factor
IL, interleukin
MAPK, mitogen-activated protein kinase
mTOR, mammalian target of rapamycin
NF, nuclear factor
PI3K, phosphatidylinositol 3-kinase
pRb, retinoblastoma protein
PTEN, phosphatase and tensin homologue deleted on chromosome 10
TNF, tumour necrosis factor
VEGF, vascular endothelial growth factor

certain malignancies.[15] This genetic expression profiling will not only be important for accurate diagnosis but also for determining prognosis and candidates for certain therapies.[16]

Another new blossoming area of research is cancer proteomics.[17] In this field, as the result of carcinogenesis, abnormalities in protein networks extend outside the cancer cell to the tissue microenvironment in which exchange of cytokines, enzymes and other proteins occurs to the advantage of the malignant cell. These molecules can be identified and become the target for new diagnostic and/or therapeutic targets. Major progress is occurring in the proteomics field in discovery of biomarkers that may be useful in predicting the clinical response to anticancer therapy.[18]

Major research advances have not only occurred during the past few years in cancer biology, genetics prevention and screening, but also in cancer treatment.[19] There is evidence of an increasing number of newer targeted therapies that can improve survival in some of the most common cancers but are also active against several other malignancies. Targeted therapy has advantages of oral administration for many agents and directed attack on cancer cells, sparing most healthy cells including the hair and bone marrow.

One of the first randomized studies carried out in hormone refractory prostate cancer cases of a cancer vaccine (APC 8015), designed to enhance a patient's immune system to attack prostate cancer cells, has shown a 17% increase in overall survival for those receiving the vaccine compared with a placebo control (25.9 months compared with 22 months).[20] Follow-up 3 years later revealed three times as many alive vs. the placebo group. Confirmation of these data by other studies is awaited. Of note, a detailed review of new and future therapeutic targets has been recently published.[21] Also, multidisciplinary treatment guidelines from the National Comprehensive Cancer Network for prostate cancer have been recently updated.[22]

The *Dana-Farber Cancer Institute atlas of diagnostic oncology* was originally published in 1991 as a comprehensive reference and teaching aid in the various clinical, laboratory, pathological and radiological features of specific cancers. Because of the recent progress in understanding the molecular biology of cancer and the development of multiple chemotherapeutic agents it became apparent that there was a need for a combination of the teaching aspects of the *Atlas* with a review and recommendations of modern therapeutic programmes available to cancer patients. Thus arose the new *Dana-Farber Cancer Institute handbooks* of four common cancers – breast, colorectal, lung and prostate. Relevant sections of the 3rd edition of the *Atlas* have been updated and are now combined with a new chapter that includes treatment strategies.

In each of our *Handbooks* the authors will review important aspects of each cancer, including epidemiology, diagnostic work-up and staging evaluation, with photographic examples of pathology subtypes and clinical presentations, followed by an up-to-date detailed discussion of multimodality treatment programmes with current recommendations where necessary. In this book on prostate cancer, Dr William Oh, Clinical

Director of the Lank Center for Genitourinary Oncology at Dana-Farber Cancer Institute, reviews various aspects of comprehensive treatment including the use of new drugs and targeted agents. The importance of patient symptom management and quality of life efforts are also addressed.

REFERENCES

1. Kamangar F, Dores GM, Anderson WF: Patterns of cancer incidence, mortality, and prevalence across five continents: defining priorities to reduce cancer disparities in different geographic regions of the world. J Clin Oncol 2006; 24(14); 2137–2150.
2. Ezzati M, Henley SJ, Lopez AD, Thun MJ: Role of smoking in global and regional cancer epidemiology: Current patterns and data needs. Int J Cancer 2005; 116: 963–971.
3. Neugent AI: Cancer epidemiology and prevention. Sci Am 2004; 12: 2–11.
4. Yancik R: Population aging and cancer: A cross-national concern. Cancer J 2005; 11: 437–441.
5. Smith RA, Cokkinides V, Eyre HJ: American Cancer Society guidelines for the early detection of cancer, 2006. Cancer J Clin 2006; 56(1): 11–25.
6. Gloeckler LA, Reichman ME, Riedel Lewis D, et al: Cancer survival and incidence from the Surveillance, Epidemiology, and End Results (SEER) program. Oncologist 2003; 8: 541–552.
7. Jemal A, Siegel R, Ward E, et al: Cancer statistics, 2006. CA Cancer J Clin 2006; 56: 106–130.
8. Jimbo M, Nease DE, Ruffin MT, et al: Information technology and cancer prevention. CA Cancer J Clin 2006; 56: 26–36.
9. Tsao AS, Kim ES, Hong WK: Chemoprevention of cancer. Cancer J Clin 2004; 54: 150–180.
10. Nelson WG, De Marzo AM, Isaacs WB: Prostate cancer. N Engl J Med 2003; 349: 366–381.
11. Thompson IM, Goodman PJ, Tangen CM, et al: The influence of finasteride on the development of prostate cancer. N Engl J Med 2003; 349: 215–224.
12. Kelloff GJ, Lippman SM, Dannenberg AJ, et al: Progress in chemoprevention drug development: The promise of molecular biomarkers for prevention of intraepithelial neoplasia and cancer – a plan to move forward. Clin Cancer Res 2006; 12(12): 3661–3697.
13. Schottenfeld D, Beebe-Dimmer J: Chronic inflammation: A common and important factor in the pathogenesis of neoplasia. CA Cancer J Clin 2006; 56: 69–83.
14. Chen Y, Hunter DJ: Molecular epidemiology of cancer. Cancer J Clin 2005; 55(1): 45–54.
15. Ramaswamy S, Golub TR: DNA microarrays in clinical oncology. J Clin Oncol 2002; 20(7): 1932–1941.
16. Quackenbush J: Microarray analysis and tumor classification. N Engl J Med 2006; 354: 2463–2472.
17. Geho DH, Petricoin EF, Liotta LA: Blasting into the microworld of tissue proteomics: A new window on cancer. Clin Cancer Research 2004; 10: 825–827.

18. Smith L, Lind MJ, Welham KJ, et al: Cancer proteomics and its application to discovery of therapy response markers in human cancer. Cancer 2006; 107(2): 232–241.

19. Herbst RS, Bajorin DF, Bleiberg H, et al: Clinical cancer advances 2005: Major research advances in cancer treatment, prevention, and screening – a report from the American Society of Clinical Oncology. J Clin Oncol 2006; 24(1): 190–205.

20. Small EJ, Schellhammer PF, et al: Immunotherapy (APC8015) for androgen independent prostate cancer (AIPC): Final survival data from a phase 3 randomized placebo-controlled trial. Orlando, FL, ASCO Prostate Cancer Symposium, February 2005.

21. Von Hoff DD, Gray PJ, Dragovich T: Pursuing therapeutic targets that are and are not there: a tumor's context of vulnerability. Sem Oncol 2006; 33(4): 367–368.

22. Scardino PT, Anscher M, Babaian RJ, et al: NCCN prostate cancer clinical practice guidelines in oncology. J Natl Compr Canc Netw 2004; 4: 224–248.

The role of molecular probes and other markers in the diagnosis and characterization of malignancy

2

Tad Wieczorek and Janina A. Longtine

Histopathological assessment is still the cornerstone in the diagnosis, classification and grading of malignancies. Light microscopic evaluation augmented by histochemical stains is sufficient in the majority of cases to provide adequate information for diagnosis and prognostication. However, it is limited by subjectivity and imprecision in the evaluation of poorly differentiated malignancies, tumours of unknown primary origin and unusual neoplasms. In an era of increasingly sophisticated therapeutic protocols (which sometimes target the molecular events leading to cancer) and the need to maximize information gained from minimally invasive samples (such as core biopsy or fine-needle aspiration), ancillary techniques have been developed to increase the specificity and reproducibility of diagnosis. These rely on cell-specific antigen expression and, more importantly, tumour-specific genetic changes that provide diagnostic, prognostic and/or therapeutic information.

In most instances, the advent of monoclonal antibodies directed against cellular proteins, coupled with the immunoperoxidase technique, has superseded direct ultrastructural evaluation in allowing more accurate designation of the epithelial, mesenchymal, haematolymphoid, neuroendocrine or glial origin of neoplasms. A cardinal example is immunolocalization of cytoskeletal intermediate filaments, which are differentially expressed in different cell types. Table 2.1 lists the intermediate filaments most useful in determining the cell lineage of tumours. The cytokeratins are a complex family of polypeptides that are expressed in various combinations in different epithelial cell types. Antibodies to cytokeratin subtypes can sometimes be utilized to identify the epithelial origin of a metastatic carcinoma of unknown primary site. For example, the pattern of reactivity for cytokeratin 7 (54 kD), which is expressed in most glandular and ductal epithelium and transitional epithelium of the urinary tract, and for cytokeratin 20 (46 kD), which is more restricted in its expression, has been helpful in this regard.[1]

In addition to the intermediate filaments, other monoclonal antibodies to cellular or tumour antigens are available. In the past decade, advances in the technique of immunohistochemistry have allowed

Table 2.1 Cytoskeletal intermediate filaments

Cell type	Intermediate filaments	Molecular weight or subtype	Presence in tumour
Epithelial	Cytokeratins	40–67	Keratinizing and non-keratinizing carcinomas
Mesenchymal	Vimentin	58	Wide distribution: sarcomas, melanomas, many lymphomas, some carcinomas
Muscle	Desmin	53	Leiomyosarcomas, rhabdomyosarcomas
Glial astrocytes	Glial fibrillary acidic protein	51	Gliomas (including astrocytomas), ependymomas
Neurons	Neurofilament proteins	68, 160, 200	Neural tumours, neuroblastomas

consistent, reliable application in routinely processed surgical pathology specimens.[2] Antigen retrieval techniques (including proteolytic digestion and heat-induced antigen retrieval), sensitive detection systems, automation and a broad range of antibodies have all contributed to this advance. Table 2.2 lists a panel of antibodies that can be utilized in routine formalin-fixed paraffin-embedded tissue to diagnose poorly differentiated neoplasms. A differential diagnosis is generated by clinical and morphological features, which can then be further refined by the use of immunohistochemistry. It is important to realize that the majority of antibodies are not entirely specific in lineage determination, and "aberrant" staining patterns are observed. In addition, there is biological variation in poorly differentiated neoplasms resulting in variation in protein expression. Therefore, accuracy is enhanced by using a panel of antisera to determine lineage or primary site. One application of this principle is distinguishing between poorly differentiated adenocarcinoma and mesothelioma in pleural tumours. Table 2.3 demonstrates the differential immunoprofile.

While a panel of monoclonal markers greatly aids in the diagnosis of a particular cancer, three malignancies can be confirmed solely by demonstrating the presence of a highly specific protein. Papillary and

Table 2.2 Immunocytochemistry in the differential diagnosis of malignancies

Malignancy	Keratin	Chromo-granin/ synaptophysin	S100	MART-1	LCA	OCT 3/4	SMA/ desmin
Carcinoma	+	−	−/+	−	−	−	−
Germ cell	+/−*	−	−	−	−	+/−	−
Lymphoma	−	−	−	−	+	−	−
Melanoma	−	−	+	+/−	−	−	−
Neuroendocrine	+/−	+	−	−	−	−	−
Sarcoma**	−/+	−	−/+	−/+	−	−	+/−

+ positive   +/− mainly positive, occasionally negative
− negative   −/+ mainly negative, occasionally positive

* Keratin is usually negative in seminomas, but positive in non-seminomatous germ cell tumours

**Sarcomas are a heterogeneous family of neoplasms and immunohistochemical staining patterns depend on the specific histological subtype

MART-1, Melanoma antigen recognized by T cells 1
LCA, Leukocyte common antigen
OCT3/4, Organic cation transporter 3/4
SMA, Smooth muscle actin

Table 2.3 Antibody panel in the differential diagnosis of adenocarcinoma and mesothelioma

Malignancy	Keratin*	WT-1	CD15 (Leu-M1)	CEA
Adenocarcinoma	+	−	+	+
Mesothelioma	+	+	−	−

*Keratin positivity in the appropriate clinicopathological setting limits the differential diagnosis to adenocarcinoma and mesothelioma

+ positive   − negative
CEA, carcinoembryonic antigen

follicular thyroid carcinomas are characterized by immunoreactivity to thyroglobulin, prostate carcinoma by detection of prostate-specific antigen, and breast carcinoma by a positive reaction for gross cystic disease fluid protein, which is present in approximately 50–70% of cases. It is noteworthy that the latter protein is also present in the rare apocrine gland carcinoma. Other antibodies which are not tissue-specific markers but useful in antibody panels include TTF-1 for pulmonary adenocarcinoma, RCC antigen for renal cell carcinoma, CD117 (c-kit) for gastrointestinal stromal tumours and CD31 (platelet endothelial cell adhesion molecule) for vascular endothelial neoplasms. Immunostains are also helpful in the delineation of normal tissue architecture and its abrogation in neoplasia. For example, immunostaining for p63 (a nuclear antigen expressed in myoepithelial cells of the breast and basal cells of the prostate) aids in the detection of ductal/glandular structures without the normal myoepithelial framework, the hallmark of invasive neoplasia.

While the cellular proteins expressed in particular types of neoplasia are fundamental to their diagnostic characterization, somatic mutations (i.e. mutations that occur in the genes of non-germline tissues) are central to the development of cancer. A series of different mutations in critical genes is probably necessary for malignant transformation to occur. The mutations may be deletions, duplications, point mutations and/or chromosomal translocations in the DNA of the tumour precursor cell. The mutations affect regulation of the cell cycle, differentiation, apoptosis, or cell–cell and cell–matrix interactions. Different neoplasms have different combinations of genetic alterations, which lead to clonal proliferations of cells. These genetic alterations, although fundamental in tumour biology, can also be used as diagnostic or prognostic markers for malignancies. This is best characterized in lymphomas and leukaemias where specific genetic translocations result in the production of chimeric mRNA and novel proteins. These translocations are the *sine qua non* for the classification of some leukaemias, such as the Philadelphia chromosome t(9;22)(q34;q11) for chronic myelogenous leukaemia and t(15;17)(q22;q11-21) for acute promyelocytic leukaemia.[3] Single nucleotide mutations may also be important in haematopoietic neoplasia; for example the *JAK2* V617F mutation is frequently present in chronic myeloproliferative disorders.[4] While genetic alterations in carcinomas are more complex than single point mutations or chromosome translocations, simple chromosomal translocations also commonly occur in (and characterize) soft tissue tumours.[5,6]

A global assessment of structural cytogenetic changes in a neoplasm is provided by full karyotypic analysis, which requires fresh, viable tumour. By contrast, fluorescence *in situ* hybridization (FISH) is a more targeted approach that can be performed on interphase nuclei obtained from frozen or fixed paraffin-embedded tissue and can identify specific characteristic cytogenetic abnormalities as an adjunct to tumour diagnosis. For example, FISH probes that flank the *EWS* gene region show a "split apart" signal when an *EWS* rearrangement is present, as in Ewing's sarcoma (see Figure 2.1). In addition, many of the characteristic cytogenetic abnormalities of neoplasms have been cloned and sequenced allowing for the utilization of molecular biology techniques such as Southern blot hybridization or, more commonly, the polymerase chain reaction (PCR). These techniques utilize fresh or frozen tumour, or even fixed, embedded tissue (with PCR), and improve diagnoses by identifying the characteristic chromosomal translocations of malignancies at the molecular level. With PCR, a specific translocation can be detected in as little as 1 in 100,000 or 1 in 1,000,000 cells as compared with 1 in 100 for FISH analysis. Thus, PCR provides a sensitive method for diagnosis and for monitoring response to therapy. For example, the t(9;22)(q34:q11) of chronic myelogenous leukaemia juxtaposes the *BCR* and *ABL1* genes resulting in a unique chimeric mRNA that can be detected by a quantitative real-time RT-PCR technique. Peripheral blood cell RNA is converted to cDNA by reverse transcription (RT). The resultant *BCR-ABL1* cDNA is quantified by monitoring fluorescently labelled oligonucleotide probes that specifically hybridize with the target during each cycle of PCR amplification (see Figure 2.2). Clinical trials with the tyrosine kinase inhibitor imatinib

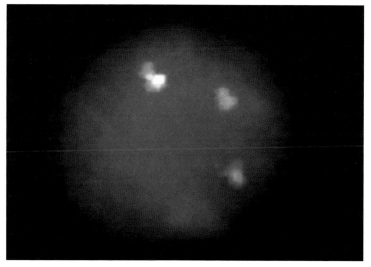

Fig. 2.1 Fluorescence *in situ* hybridization (FISH) on a sample obtained by fine-needle aspiration shows an interphase nucleus with red and green probes flanking each of two copies of the *EWS* gene, demonstrating one fused and one split signal. The split signal indicates rearrangement of the *EWS* gene region. (Courtesy of Dr. Paola Dal Cin, Cytogenetics Laboratory, Brigham and Women's Hospital.)

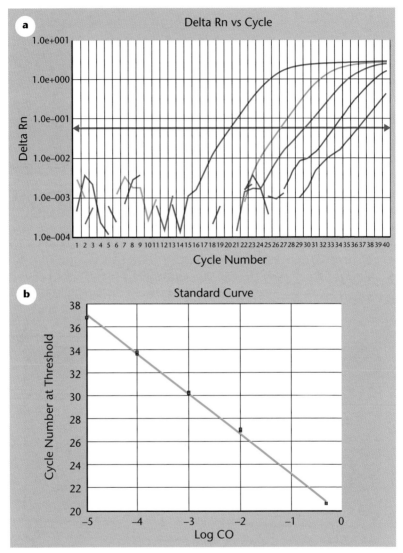

Fig. 2.2 (a) "Taq-Man™" (Applied Biosystems) quantitative RT-PCR results for dilutions (1:1,10^{-2}, 10^{-3}, 10^{-4}, 10^{-5}) of K562 cell line RNA which express chimeric *BCR-ABL1* mRNA. After approximately 15 cycles of PCR, the sample with the most *BCR-ABL1* mRNA (1:1) enters the linear phase of exponential amplification as measured by fluorescence accumulation monitored in real time. Samples with less target require more PCR cycles to reach the exponential phase. (b) For quantitation, a standard curve is generated plotting the PCR cycle number at threshold (red line in middle of exponential phase) against log concentration of target. Unknown samples can be quantified by plotting against the standard curve.

defined a target of a minimal residual level of *BCR-ABL1* RNA transcripts that is associated with progression-free survival (see Figure 2.3).[7,8] Rising levels of *BCR-ABL1* mRNA in patients on tyrosine kinase inhibitors or status post transplantation are indicative of a molecular relapse and the need for alternate or additional therapy. Southern blot hybridization or PCR can also identify clonal rearrangements of the immunoglobulin or T-cell receptor genes as an adjunct to the diagnosis of lymphoma or lymphoid leukaemias (see Figure 2.4).

Genetic analysis of neoplasms may also provide prognostic information, such as identifying the *BCR-ABL1* rearrangement in Philadelphia chromosome-positive acute lymphoblastic leukaemia (ALL) or *N-MYC* amplification in neuroblastoma. In addition, genetic analysis is playing an increasing role in therapeutic planning, as therapies tailored to specific genetic "lesions" are developed. Examples of such lesions include *HER2* amplification in breast cancer[9] and the epidermal growth factor receptor gene (*EGFR*) mutation in lung cancer.[10,11] These genetic lesions

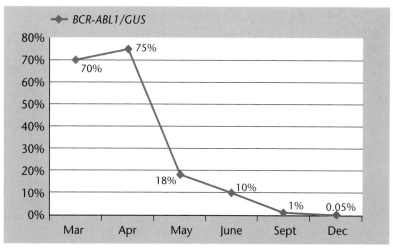

Fig. 2.3 Timeline of response to the tyrosine kinase inhibitor imatinib as monitored by real-time RT-PCR analysis of *BCR-ABL1* mRNA expressed as a ratio to the normalizing gene, *GUS*. Patients who achieve a 3-log reduction of transcript level by 12 months of therapy have a negligible risk of disease progression in the following 12 months.[8]

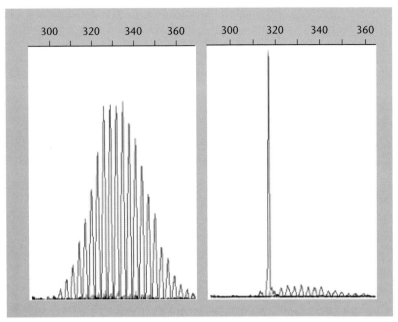

Fig. 2.4 Polymerase chain reaction (PCR) amplification of the immunoglobulin heavy chain (IgH) gene with primers to the variable and joining regions that flank the unique IgH gene rearrangement of B-cells. B-cell IgH rearrangements differ by size and sequence. Fluorescent primers are incorporated into the PCR product, which are then analyzed by capillary gel electrophoresis. (a) The Gaussian distribution of a polyclonal population of B cells. (b) A dominant peak of 318 bp representing a monoclonal population in a B-cell lymphoma.

may be detected either by evaluation of aberrant protein expression (as in immunohistochemical detection of membranous overexpression of HER2 oncoprotein in breast cancer), by gene amplification (as in FISH analysis of *HER2*), or by molecular testing (as in *EGFR* point or small deletion mutation analysis in lung cancer, see Figure 2.5). Quantification of the expression levels of large numbers of genes in specific types of neoplasia by oligonucleotide chips or cDNA microarrays, "expression profiling", has led to the identification of subsets of genes that provide prognostic information, such as in diffuse large B-cell lymphoma (see Figure 2.6).[12] It has even become feasible to measure the expression level of multiple genes (by RT-PCR) in routinely prepared, paraffin-embedded tumour samples, as in the multigene assay to

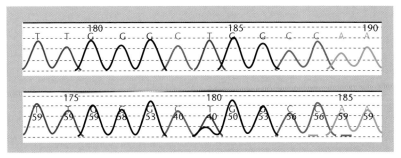

Fig. 2.5 Lung adenocarcinoma DNA sequence analysis of exon 21 of the *EGFR* receptor gene. The top row shows normal or wildtype exon sequence. The bottom row shows the heterozygous T to C point mutation, which characterizes the L858R mutation, a common mutation in carcinomas responsive to tyrosine kinase inhibitors.

predict recurrence of tamoxifen-treated, node-negative breast cancer.[13] This assay measures the expression level of genes involved in key aspects of tumour biology such as proliferation, invasion and oestrogen response and its quantitative result has potential application in therapeutic planning. As key genes (and hence proteins) are identified by expression profiling, expression can be assayed by routine immunohistochemistry. An important and practical example of this strategy was the development of a specific antibody to P504S (AMACR/racemase), a protein product strongly expressed in prostatic adenocarcinoma and prostatic intraepithelial neoplasia, but typically not in benign prostatic epithelium.[14] This immunostain is therefore useful in supporting a diagnosis of prostatic adenocarcinoma in cases where the morphological findings are subtle – as in the diagnosis of minimal adenocarcinoma on needle biopsy.

The genetics of cancer also extends to inherited predisposition to neoplasms described in a number of families.[15] These syndromes include germline mutations of tumour suppressor genes, such as familial retinoblastoma, and mutations of DNA repair genes as in ataxiatelangectasia or hereditary non-polyposis colon cancer. Some of these are listed in Table 2.4.

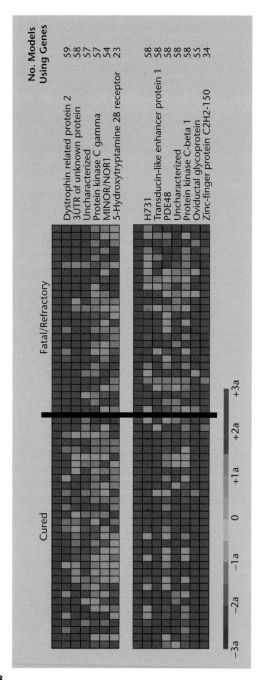

Fig. 2.6 Genes included in the DLBCL outcome model. Genes expressed at higher levels in cured disease are listed on top and those that were more abundant in fatal disease are shown on the bottom. Red indicates high expression; blue, low expression. Colour scale at bottom indicates relative expression in standard deviations from the mean. Each column is a sample, each row is a gene. Expression profiles of the 32 cured DLBCLs are on the left; profiles of the fatal/refractory tumours are on the right. Models with the highest accuracy were obtained using 13 genes. Reproduced by permission from Macmillan Publishers Ltd: Nature Medicine. Shipp M, Ross K, Tamayo P, et al: Diffuse large B-cell lymphoma outcome prediction by gene expression profiling and supervised machine learning. Nature Med 2002; 8: 68–74. © 2002.

Table 2.4 Examples of inherited syndromes predisposing to cancer

Syndrome	Chromosome locus	Gene
Ataxia-telangiactasia	11q22	*ATM*
Hereditary breast/ovarian cancer	17q21	*BRCA1*
	13q12	*BRCA2*
Familial adenomatous polyposis	5q21-q22	*APC*
Familial retinoblastoma	13q14	*RB1*
Hereditary non-polyposis colorectal cancer (Lynch syndrome)	2p22-p21	*MSH2*
	3p21	*MLH1*
	2q31-q33	*PMS1*
	7p22	*PMS2*
Li-Fraumeni	17p13	*TP53*
Multiple endocrine neoplasia, Type 1	11q13	*MEN1*
Multiple endocrine neoplasia, Type 2	10q11.2	*RET*
Neurofibromatosis, Type 1	17q11	*NF1*
Neurofibromatosis, Type 2	22q12	*NF2*
von Hippel-Lindau disease	3p26-p25	*VHL*

REFERENCES

1. Chu P, Wu E, Weiss LM: Cytokeratin 7 and cytokeratin 20 expression in epithelial neoplasms: a survey of 435 cases. Mod Pathol 2000; 13(9): 962–971.
2. Chan JKC: Advances in immunohistochemistry: Impact on surgical pathology practice. Seminars Diagn Pathol 2000; 17: 170–177.
3. Jaffe ES, Stein HN, Vardiman JW, eds: World Health Organization Classification of Tumours, Pathology and Genetics of Tumours of Haematopoietic and Lymphoid Tissues. IARC Press, Lyon, 2001.
4. Percy MJ, McMullin MF: The V617F JAK2 mutation and the myeloproliferative disorders. Hematol Oncol 2005; 23(3-4): 91–93.
5. Sandberg AA: Cytogenetics and molecular genetics of bone and soft-tissue tumors. Am J Med Genet 2002; 115(3): 189–193.
6. Antonescu CR: The role of genetic testing in soft tissue sarcoma. Histopathology 2006; 48(1): 13–21.
7. O'Brien SG, Guilhot F, Larson RA, et al: Imatinib compared with interferon and low-dose cytarabine for newly diagnosed chronic-phase chronic myeloid leukemia. N Engl J Med 2003; 348: 994–1004.
8. Hughes TP, Kaeda J, Branford S, et al: Frequency of major molecular responses to imatinib or interferon alfa plus cytarabine in newly diagnosed chronic myeloid leukemia. N Engl J Med 2003; 349: 1423–1432.

9. Slamon DJ, Leyland-Jones B, Shak S, et al: Use of chemotherapy plus a monoclonal antibody against HER2 for metastatic breast cancer that overexpresses HER2. N Engl J Med 2001; 344: 783–792.

10. Lynch TJ, Bell DW, Sordella R, et al: Activating mutations in the epidermal growth factor receptor underlying responsiveness of non-small-cell lung cancer to gefitinib. N Engl J Med 2004; 350: 2129–2139.

11. Paez JG, Janne PA, Lee JC, et al: EGFR mutations in lung cancer: correlation with clinical response to gefitinib therapy. Science 2004; 304: 1497–1500.

12. Shipp M, Ross K, Tamayo P, et al: Diffuse large B-cell lymphoma outcome prediction by gene expression profiling and supervised machine learning. Nature Med 2002; 8: 68–74.

13. Paik S, Shak S, Tang G, et al: A multigene assay to predict recurrence of tamoxifen-treated, node-negative breast cancer. N Engl J Med 2004; 351: 2817–2826.

14. Beach R, Gown AM, De Peralta-Venturina MN, et al: P504S immunohistochemical detection in 405 prostatic specimens including 376 18-gauge needle biopsies. Am J Surg Pathol 2002; 26(12): 1588–1596.

15. Scriver CR, Beaudet AL, Sly WS, Valle D, eds: Metabolic and Molecular Bases of Inherited Disease, 8th edn. McGraw-Hill, New York, 2001.

Prostate cancer: epidemiology, histology, diagnosis and staging

3

Robert W. Ross, Mari Nakabayashi, Marc B. Garnick, Christopher L. Corless, Philip W. Kantoff, William K. Oh

Prostate cancer is the most commonly diagnosed non-cutaneous malignancy in men in the US. In 2007, over 218,000 cases will be diagnosed and over 27,000 men will die of the disease. The incidence of prostate cancer increased rapidly in the early 1990s because of the widespread use of the prostate-specific antigen (PSA) test, but subsequently levelled off in the late 1990s. Mortality from prostate cancer has also begun to decline recently, though the cause for this drop is not known.

The incidence of prostate cancer increases rapidly with age, particularly after the age of 50, although the presence of pathological prostate cancer in men less than 50 years of age has been demonstrated in autopsy series. Age, race and family history are the most well-established risk factors for prostate cancer. Scandinavians, Americans, and particularly African Americans, have a very high incidence of prostate cancer compared with Asian men. Diet may also be important. The results of studies including men who migrate from areas of low incidence to areas of high incidence and acquire intermediate probabilities of developing prostate cancer suggest that environmental factors contribute to these differences. One such factor may be the high-fat diet of the Western developed world. Another potential risk factor may be serum hormone levels, particularly testosterone, although such data are controversial. Recent data from a clinical trial of chemoprevention of prostate cancer with an inhibitor of 5-alpha reductase (the enzyme that converts testosterone to dihydrotestosterone) support the idea that alterations of the androgen milieu can alter the short-term risk of the development of prostate cancer.

A subset of patients who develop prostate cancer probably do so on the basis of genetic predisposition. Familial prostate cancer may be an important factor among patients who develop prostate cancer at a young age. First-degree relatives of men with prostate cancer have a 2–3 fold increased risk of developing prostate cancer compared with the general population. Such data have lead to a search for genetic loci that confer an increased risk of prostate cancer, including one on the long arm of chromosome 1 called HPC1. Many studies are now evaluating potential candidate genes within this locus, including *RNASEL*, an enzyme that regulates cell proliferation.

HISTOLOGY

The vast majority of prostate cancers are adenocarcinomas. Most exhibit acinar-type differentiation, but some also have features of ductal differentiation. Pure large duct prostatic adenocarcinomas are uncommon. Typical prostatic adenocarcinomas may contain foci of mucinous differentiation or neuroendocrine differentiation but the prognostic significance of these features remains uncertain. Small cell undifferentiated carcinoma of the prostate is rare but when present is often associated with areas of adenocarcinoma. Whether presenting in pure form or intermixed with adenocarcinoma, small cell undifferentiated carcinoma in the prostate carries a grave prognosis. Other tumours occurring in the prostate include transitional cell carcinoma (most often by invasion from the urethra), sarcomas of stromal origin and metastases from other organs.

The putative precursor of invasive adenocarcinoma is prostatic intraepithelial neoplasia (PIN), in which cytologically dysplastic cells are found lining normal ducts and acini. PIN is divided into low and high grades; however, only the latter is geographically associated with invasive adenocarcinoma. Although the natural history of PIN is unknown, many foci of high-grade PIN demonstrate partial loss of the basal cell layer and a transition to small invasive glands is occasionally observed. A diagnosis of high-grade PIN on needle biopsy should prompt additional studies to rule out invasive tumour.

Small foci of adenocarcinoma are found incidentally at autopsy in more than 30% of men over the age of 50 who die of unrelated causes. Thus, there is a large pool of these so-called latent or 'autopsy' prostate cancers present in the older male population. Whether clinical cancers arise from latent tumours or develop by an independent pathway is unknown.

Although a variety of grading schemes for prostate cancer have been developed, the most widely used in the US is the Gleason grading system, which is based strictly upon architectural rather than cytological features of the cancer. According to this scheme, the pattern of infiltrating tumour glands is assigned a grade from 1 (well differentiated) to 5 (poorly differentiated). Since many adenocarcinomas exhibit more than one pattern, the grades for the two most common patterns present in a tumour are added together to give a Gleason sum or Gleason score. The prognostic utility of the Gleason grading system has been validated in numerous studies wherein patients diagnosed with low Gleason score cancers have an excellent prognosis, while those with high Gleason score cancers have a poor prognosis. The main shortcoming of the Gleason grading system is that the majority of cancers are intermediate in grade. Less than 30% of cancers in most studies are within the Gleason score 2–4 or 8–10 groups. As a result, the Gleason score provides little prognostic information in most cases.

Tissue staining for PSA has become an important adjunct to confirming the diagnosis of prostate cancer. This is particularly useful in poorly differentiated cancers or those cancers that manifest themselves initially at metastatic sites as poorly differentiated carcinoma.

DIAGNOSIS AND STAGING OF PROSTATE CANCER

The detection of prostate cancer has been greatly enhanced by the introduction of the PSA test. Optimal detection of prostate cancer is now achieved through the combination of the digital rectal examination (DRE) and PSA. Biopsies are facilitated by transrectal ultrasound, which enables the physician to locate the areas of abnormality. The morbidity from biopsy is now minimal with the use of spring-loaded biopsy guns. Optimal information is acquired when multiple specially coordinated biopsies are performed. With such biopsies, the grade of the cancer, the number of cores positive for cancer and percentage of cancer per core should be determined.

A bone scan should be performed after the diagnosis of prostate cancer is made, particularly in men with a PSA in excess of 20 ng/ml or high Gleason grade disease (Gleason scores of 8–10). Although the incidence of radiographically detected regional lymph nodes is quite low, scanning by computed tomography or magnetic resonance imaging (MRI) should be considered, particularly in patients with high-grade, high-stage cancers or those patients with high PSA serum levels. Recent techniques with newer MRI contrast agents (lymphotrophic nanoparticle-enhanced MRI) may help identify regional lymph node involvement. Endorectal coil MRI should be performed at experienced centres in patients being considered for radical prostatectomy in whom the extent of local disease needs to be assessed. With the widespread use of PSA, the proportion of localized prostate cancers has increased.

Approximately 80% of cancers arising in the prostate gland arise in the peripheral zones, while 20% arise in the periuretheral or transition zone. Cancers arising in the transition zone have traditionally been diagnosed by transurethral resection of the prostate. However, with increasing use of PSA and medical therapies for benign prostatic hyperplasia (BPH), the frequency of cancers diagnosed in this manner has diminished.

Two systems are commonly used for staging of prostate cancer – the Whitmore-Jewett system (stages A through D) and the American Joint

Committee on Cancer (AJCC) tumour/node/metastases (TNM) system, last modified in 2002 (see Table 3.1). The AJCC TNM system is used more commonly now.

The majority of cancers that are currently diagnosed are detected as a result of an abnormal PSA, an abnormal DRE or both. Organ-confined, palpable cancers are classified as T2. Cancers diagnosed strictly on the basis of an abnormal PSA with no associated palpable abnormality are currently classified as T1c. Cancers that on physical examination extend into the seminal vesicles or palpably exceed beyond the prostate are categorized as T3 cancers. Stage IV cancers are those that have metastasized either to regional lymph nodes – N1 – or distant lymph nodes, bone or viscera – M1 (see Table 3.1).

Careful examination of the prostate following its removal at the time of radical prostatectomy provides critical prognostic information. There is good correlation between the grade of cancer found at the time of biopsy and that found at the time of radical prostatectomy; when discrepancy occurs the biopsies most frequently undergrade the cancer. With careful examination of the prostate, the volume of cancer can be ascertained. Similarly, vascular or perineural invasion can be ascertained, as can the degree of local extension. Cancers that are confined within the capsule are less likely to recur than those that invade through the capsule or into the seminal vesicle or demonstrate positive margins. Clinically localized tumours are frequently upstaged into T3 cancers pathologically. The frequency of lymph node involvement at the time of radical prostatectomy has apparently decreased in recent years, perhaps in part due to the more careful selection of surgical patients afforded by the use of the PSA.

CLINICAL MANIFESTATIONS

Most patients diagnosed with prostate cancer are asymptomatic and the diagnosis is made as a result of an abnormal PSA or DRE. Since the prevalence of BPH in the population of men susceptible to prostate cancer is high, many men will manifest mild degrees of prostatism. With locally advanced prostate cancer, urinary obstruction may occur, as may haematospermia. Carcinoma should be considered when obstructive urinary symptomatology develops over a short period of time. Some patients initially present with symptoms of metastatic disease either from painful bony metastasis or from lymphadenopathy. In such patients, immunostaining for PSA may be of particular value in distinguishing a carcinoma of prostatic origin.

Table 3.1 Clinical staging of prostate cancer, using the 2002 AJCC TNM classification and the Whitmore-Jewett system
Note that for patients who are post-prostatectomy, a pathological T stage is often employed (pT) in which there is no pT1 designation

2002 AJCC	Stage		Whitmore Jewett	
T1a	I	Microscopic tumour in ≤5% of prostatic chips	A	Non-palpable tumour, detected incidentally
T1b	II	Microscopic tumour in > 5% of prostatic chips		
T1c		Non-palpable tumour identified by needle biopsy	B	Palpable tumour, confined within the prostate, or detected by prostate-specific antigen
T2a		Tumour confined within the prostate, involves one half of one lobe or less		
T2b		Tumour confined within the prostate, involves more than one half of one lobe, but not both lobes		
T2c		Tumour confined within the prostate, involves both lobes		
T3a	III	Tumour extends through the prostate capsule	C	Tumour extends through the prostate capsule
T3b		Tumour invades the seminal vesicle		
T4	IV	Tumour is fixed or invades adjacent structures other than the seminal vesicle		
N1		Metastasis in regional lymph node	D1	Metastatic disease to regional lymph nodes or distant sites
M1a		Non-regional lymph node metastasis	D2	Metastasis to distant lymph nodes, bone or other sites
M1b		Bone metastasis		
M1c		Other sites		

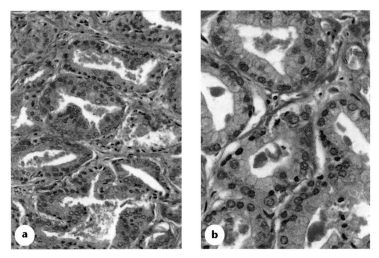

Fig. 3.1 Adenomatous hyperplasia. (**a**) In this atypical example, small, irregular, closely packed glands form a circumscribed nodule. (**b**) At higher power, the epithelial cells lack the prominent nucleoli of adenocarcinoma. A two-cell layer is present focally. Distinction of atypical adenomatous hyperplasia from well-differentiated adenocarcinoma may be difficult.

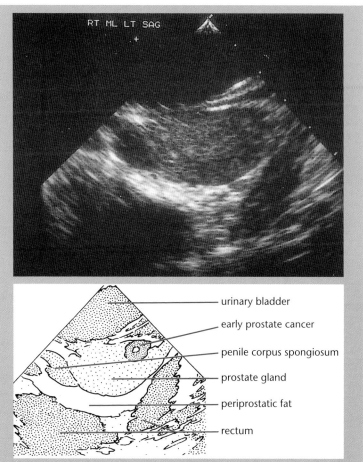

Fig. 3.2 Prostate cancer. Sagittal ultrasonogram demonstrates hypoechoic areas, which are the most common abnormalities seen with prostate cancer. Needle biopsy of hypoechoic lesions can be performed directly under ultrasonographic guidance.

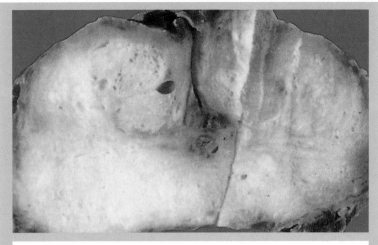

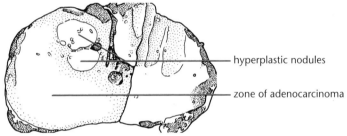

hyperplastic nodules

zone of adenocarcinoma

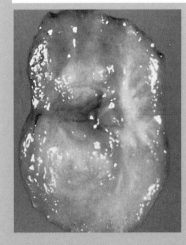

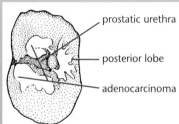

prostatic urethra

posterior lobe

adenocarcinoma

Fig. 3.3 Adenocarcinoma. (**a**) Many prostatic carcinomas arise in the posterior portion of the gland. Cystic areas in this specimen represent zones of nodular hyperplasia unrelated to the carcinoma. This site of origin is not invariably the case, however. (**b**) A yellow zone of colouration in the periurethral region in this specimen corresponds to a lesion involving both lateral lobes.

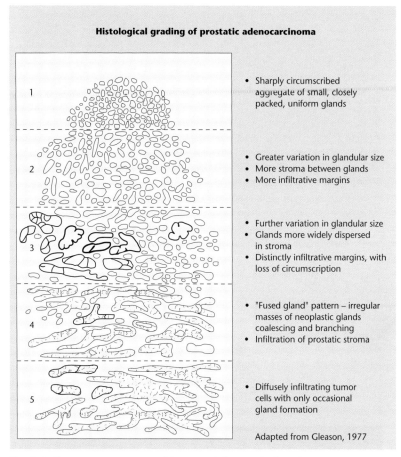

Histological grading of prostatic adenocarcinoma

1
- Sharply circumscribed aggregate of small, closely packed, uniform glands

2
- Greater variation in glandular size
- More stroma between glands
- More infiltrative margins

3
- Further variation in glandular size
- Glands more widely dispersed in stroma
- Distinctly infiltrative margins, with loss of circumscription

4
- "Fused gland" pattern – irregular masses of neoplastic glands coalescing and branching
- Infiltration of prostatic stroma

5
- Diffusely infiltrating tumor cells with only occasional gland formation

Adapted from Gleason, 1977

Fig. 3.4 Gleason pattern scores. This is one of the standard grading systems for prostate adenocarcinomas. Five histological patterns are identified. Patterns 1 and 2 correspond to well-differentiated cancers. Pattern 3 marks a moderately differentiated cancer and patterns 4 and 5 correspond to poorly differentiated or anaplastic lesions.

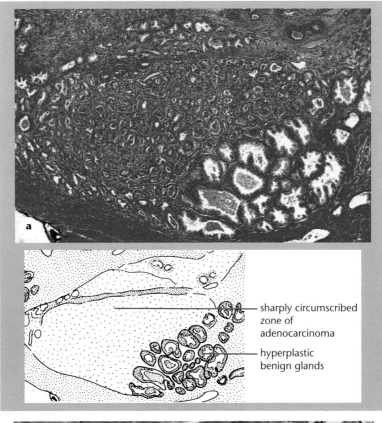

sharply circumscribed zone of adenocarcinoma

hyperplastic benign glands

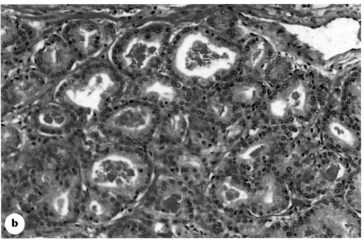

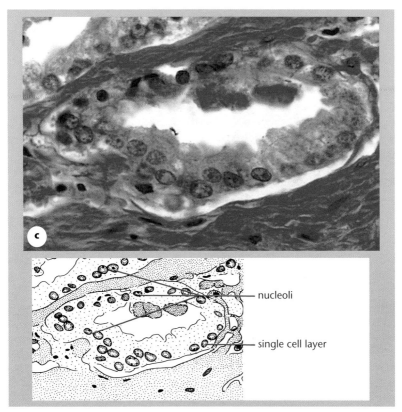

Fig. 3.5 Adenocarcinoma (Gleason grade 1). (**a**) This lesion forms a sharply circumscribed aggregate of small, uniform glands. At this magnification, distinction from atypical adenomatous hyperplasia is not possible. The larger surrounding glands are hyperplastic. (**b**) Small, uniform, closely spaced glands are the hallmark of this low-grade malignancy. Note the sharply circumscribed border, with the surrounding stroma at the top left of the field. Intraluminal crystalloids are also present. (**c**) The presence of large nucleoli in the glandular cells has been used to distinguish low-grade carcinoma from atypical adenomatous hyperplasia. This admittedly arbitrary distinction has little if any biological importance.

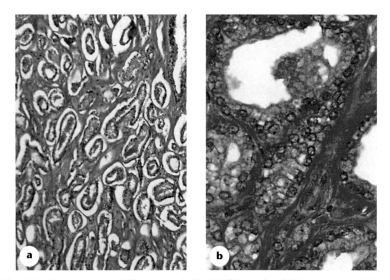

Fig. 3.6 Adenocarcinoma (Gleason grade 2). (**a**) This grade exhibits greater variation in glandular size, more stroma between glands and a more infiltrative margin than the much less common grade 1 pattern. Distinction of grade 2 lesions from grade 3 is somewhat subjective. (**b**) Carcinomatous glands are composed of a single layer of cells. The nuclei are enlarged and have prominent nucleoli.

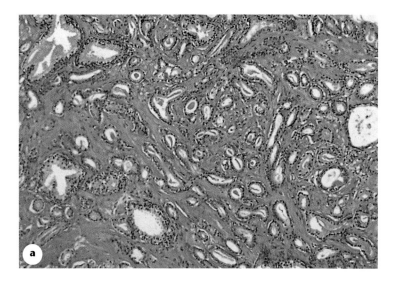

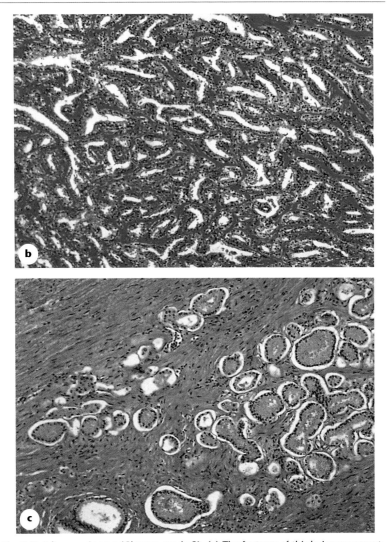

Fig. 3.7 Adenocarcinoma (Gleason grade 3). (**a**) The features of this lesion represent an extension of the changes seen in the grade 2 pattern. The glands are even more irregular in size and shape. The tumour is distinctly infiltrative, without any of the circumscription characterizing grade 1 and 2 lesions. (**b**) Glandular size and shape in this example are markedly irregular. (**c**) Diffuse infiltration of single, irregular glands is evident. Small foci such as these are commonly encountered in needle biopsy specimens.

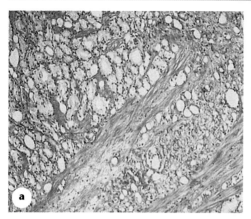

Fig. 3.8 Adenocarcinoma (Gleason grade 4). (**a**) The most common grade 4 variant of prostatic adenocarcinoma is the fused-gland pattern seen here. Back-to-back glands without intervening stroma infiltrate the prostate. (**b**) Higher-power view shows back-to-back glands infiltrating the stroma. (**c**) In another example of the fused-gland pattern, the carcinoma grows as an infiltrating sheet of cells containing scattered lumina.

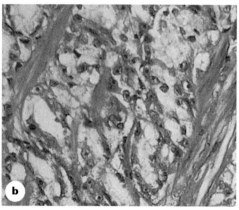

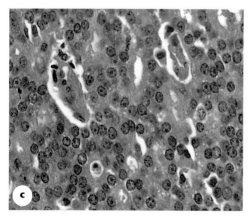

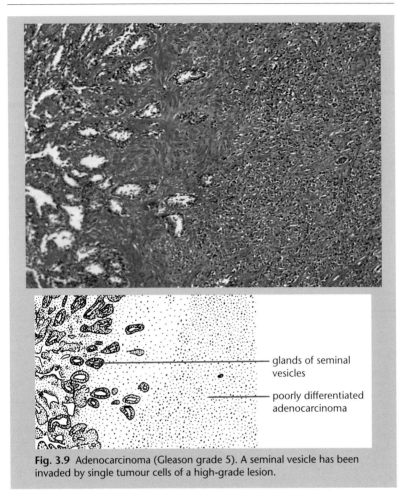

Fig. 3.9 Adenocarcinoma (Gleason grade 5). A seminal vesicle has been invaded by single tumour cells of a high-grade lesion.

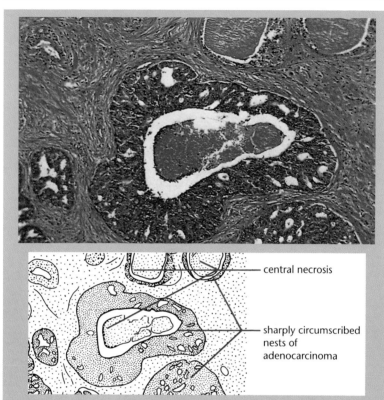

central necrosis

sharply circumscribed nests of adenocarcinoma

Fig. 3.10 Adenocarcinoma (Gleason grade 5). This lesion exhibits a comedocarcinomatous pattern. Circumscribed nests of tumour cells are similar to those seen at low power in the cribriform variant of Gleason grade 3. The presence of a central area of necrosis distinguishes this pattern from grade 3. The cells of this variant have pleomorphic, vesicular nuclei.

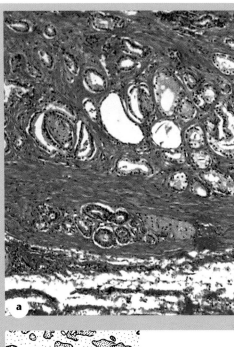

Fig. 3.11
Adenocarcinoma. (a) Glands of tumour cells have extended into the capsule but have not penetrated to the pericapsular fat.

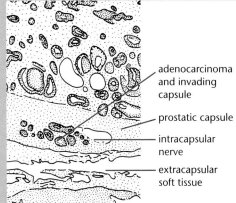

adenocarcinoma and invading capsule

prostatic capsule

intracapsular nerve

extracapsular soft tissue

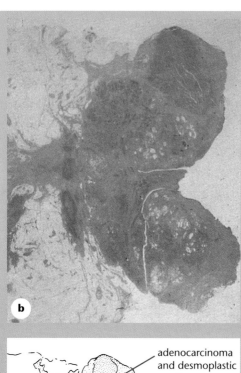

Fig. 3.11 *Continued*
Adenocarcinoma. (b) In
this instance, the lesion has
extended through the
prostatic capsule and into
the surrounding fat,
evoking a desmoplastic
reaction, which is easily
palpable on rectal
examination.

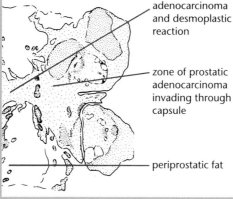

adenocarcinoma
and desmoplastic
reaction

zone of prostatic
adenocarcinoma
invading through
capsule

periprostatic fat

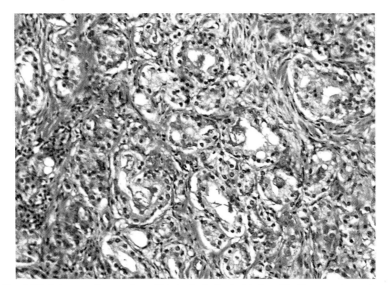

Fig. 3.12 Adenocarcinoma. Even histologically typical lesions like the one shown here often stain positively (red) with the mucicarmine technique, in contrast to normal or hyperplastic prostatic tissue. This stain may, therefore, be valuable as an adjunct to diagnosis.

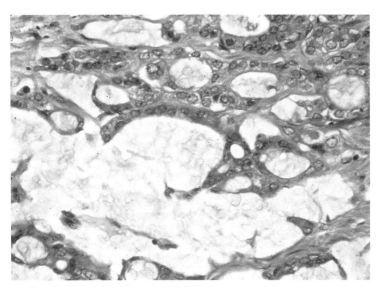

Fig. 3.13 Adenocarcinoma. Some prostatic adenocarcinomas produce abundant extracellular mucin which forms large pools in the stroma, separating tumour cells. Such carcinomas are not readily amenable to Gleason grading and may be confused with metastases from a primary gastrointestinal tumour.

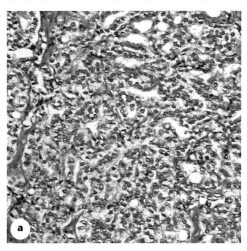

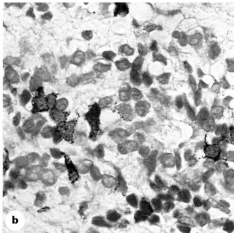

Fig. 3.14 Carcinoid-like tumour. (**a**) Nests of cells with uniform nuclei show a glandular-trabecular growth pattern resembling gastrointestinal carcinoid tumours. (**b**) Argyrophil stain demonstrates many positive (brown) cells in a prostatic carcinoid-like tumour, confirming its neuroendocrine differentiation (Churukian–Schenk stain).

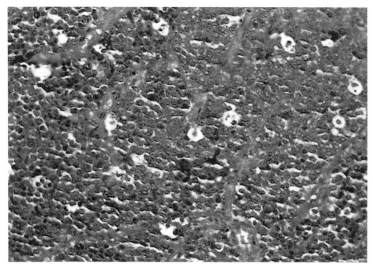

Fig. 3.15 Small cell carcinoma. Carcinomas indistinguishable by light microscopy from pulmonary small cell (oat cell) carcinoma occasionally arise in the prostate. They are usually seen in association with areas of more conventional adenocarcinoma.

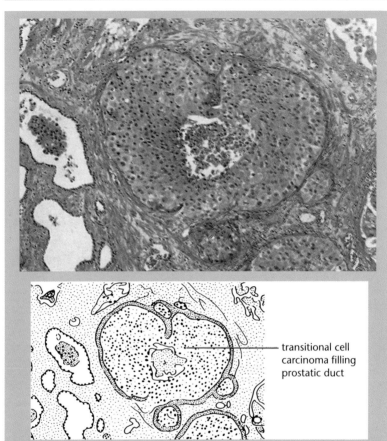

transitional cell carcinoma filling prostatic duct

Fig. 3.16 Transitional cell carcinoma. This tumour may arise in the prostatic ducts or may extend into the ducts from an initial focus in the prostatic urethra. Cytologically identical to analogous lesions of the bladder and urethra, it is characteristically composed of highly pleomorphic cells without any evidence of squamous or glandular differentiation. The closely packed, irregular contour of the tumour nests and the surrounding fibroplastic stromal reaction suggest that this is an invasive lesion rather than an *in situ* change in normal ducts.

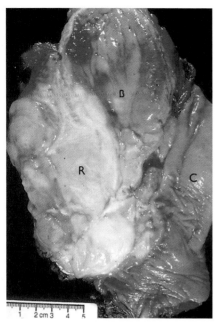

Fig. 3.17 Rhabdomyosarcoma. The tumour forms a large, fleshy mass that replaces the prostate gland and invades the bladder and signmoid colon. R, rhabdomyosarcoma replacing prostate gland; B, urinary bladder; C, distal sigmoid colon.

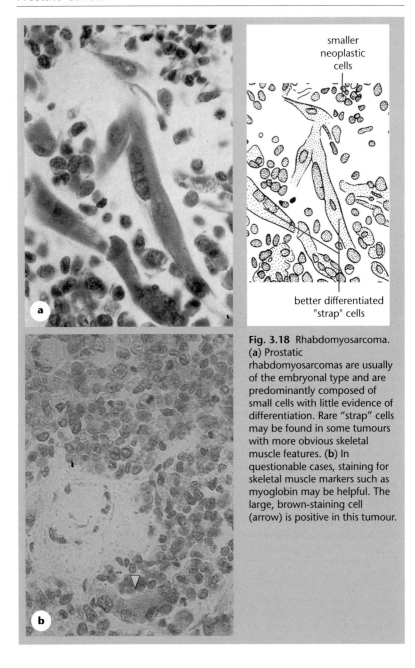

smaller
neoplastic
cells

better differentiated
"strap" cells

Fig. 3.18 Rhabdomyosarcoma. (a) Prostatic rhabdomyosarcomas are usually of the embryonal type and are predominantly composed of small cells with little evidence of differentiation. Rare "strap" cells may be found in some tumours with more obvious skeletal muscle features. (b) In questionable cases, staining for skeletal muscle markers such as myoglobin may be helpful. The large, brown-staining cell (arrow) is positive in this tumour.

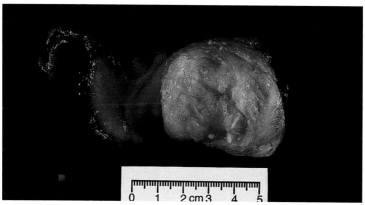

Fig. 3.19 Leiomyosarcoma of prostate. Leiomyosarcoma of prostate, although rare (comprising less than 0.1% of primary prostatic neoplasms), is the single most common prostatic sarcoma typically occurring in older adults (26% of cases). The tumour is characterized by fascicular arrangements of spindle-shaped cells with brightly eosinophilic cytoplasm and strong immunohistochemical positivity for smooth muscle actin and weaker positivity for desmin. Precise criteria for distinction from (benign) leiomyoma have not been proven reliable. Reactive myofibroblastic/fibroblastic proliferations such as a postoperative spindle cell nodule should also be considered in the differential diagnosis.

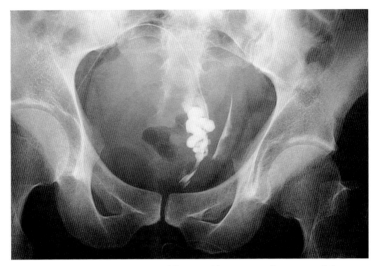

Fig. 3.20 Prostate sarcoma. 35-year-old man with an unusual sarcoma of the prostate. Vasogram shows dilated seminal vesicle due to obstruction from the tumour.

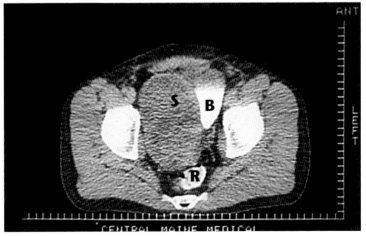

Fig. 3.21 Prostate sarcoma. Same patient. CT scan shows large sarcoma of the prostate (S) displacing the urinary bladder (B) and rectum (R).

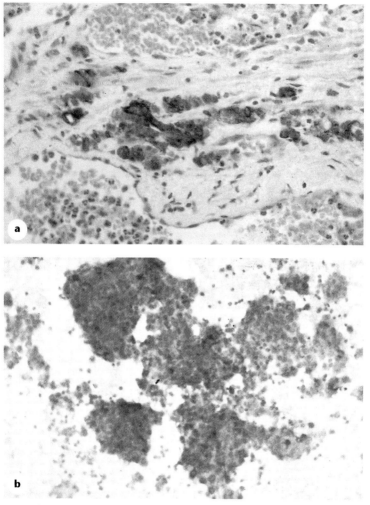

Fig. 3.22 Metastatic adenocarcinoma of prostate. (a) This biopsy specimen containing a high-grade adenocarcinoma stains positively for anti-prostate-specific antigen (PSA), strongly supporting a prostatic origin. (b) Antibodies directed against PSA and prostatic acid phosphatase in this needle aspiration cytology specimen of lung tissue react positively for the latter, indicating a prostatic origin.

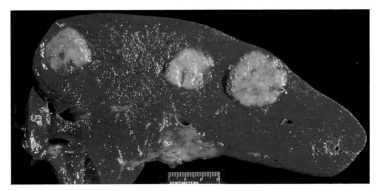

Fig. 3.23 Liver metastases. In unusual instances, prostate cancer can metastasize to the liver. Discrete nodularity is the most common pattern. (Courtesy of Pathology Department, Brigham and Women's Hospital, Boston, MA.)

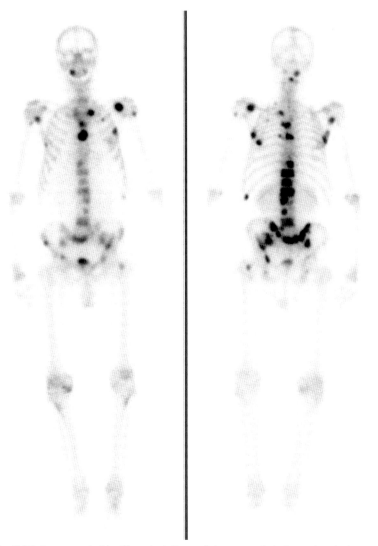

Fig. 3.24 Bone scan to identify metastatic prostate cancer. Anterior and posterior view of a bone scan of a patient with multiple bony metastases from his prostate cancer. This pattern is typical for prostate cancer, with involvement of the thoracic and lumbar spine and bilateral hips, with relative sparing of the long bones of the extremities.

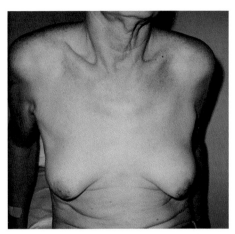

Fig. 3.25 Gynaecomastia in a man treated with diethylstilbestrol (DES) for advanced prostate cancer. As oestrogenic therapies (including the herbal therapy PC-SPES) are now being increasingly used for androgen-independent prostate cancer, recognition of this complication is important. In addition, antiandrogen monotherapy can also lead to significant gynaecomastia. A short course of prophylactic breast irradiation may inhibit growth of breast tissue.

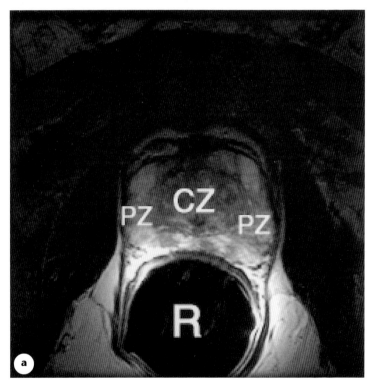

Fig. 3.26 Two axial T2 weighted images from a prostate MRI using an endorectal coil. (a) At a relatively superior level in the prostate, the normal differentiation between the lower signal central zone (CZ) and the higher signal peripheral zone (PZ) is evident. The rectum (R) is distended by the coil.

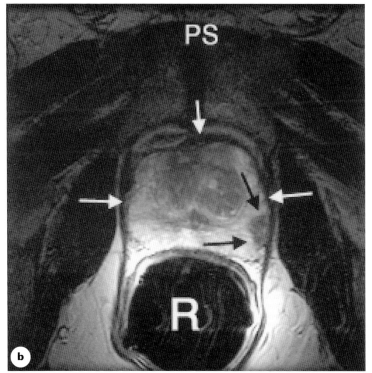

Fig. 3.26 *Continued* (**b**) At a lower position in the prostate, a focal area of low signal in the left peripheral zone is seen (black arrows), indicating an area of infiltration with tumour. The margins of the prostate capsule (white arrows) appear intact. The rectum (R) and pubic symphysis (PS) are marked for orientation.

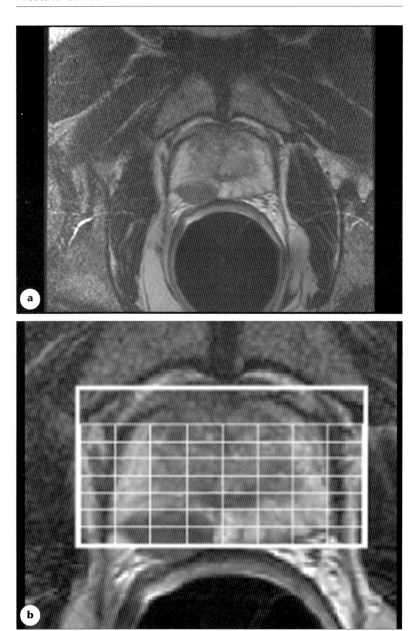

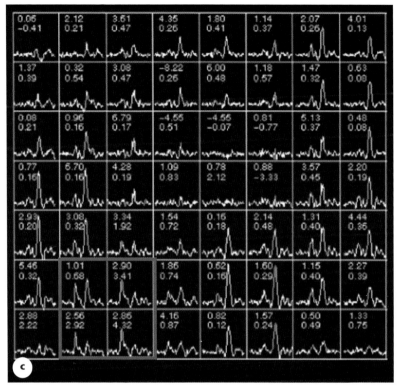

Fig. 3.27 Magnetic resonance spectroscopy to identify prostate cancer. (**a**) T2 weighted endorectal MRI imaging revealing an abnormal region of hypointensity within the right aspect of the peripheral zone of the prostate gland. (**b**) Superimposed upon the T2 weighted image is the localized spectroscopic volume of investigation. Within each voxel the choline and citrate spectrum are investigated. (**c**) Localized spectra from each voxel. Voxels that are suspicious for cancer demonstrate increased choline (the first peak on the left) and decreased citrate peaks (highlighted). (Courtesy of Dr. Fergus Coakley, University of California, San Francisco.)

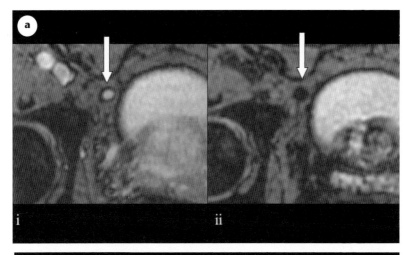

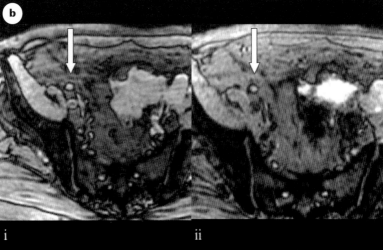

Fig. 3.28 Lymphotropic nanoparticle-enhanced MRI to identify involved lymph nodes. (a) (i) T2* weighted endorectal MRI image at the level of the acetabulum pre-iron oxide nanoparticle contrast displaying a normally enhancing external iliac node. (ii) Post-iron oxide nanoparticle contrast T2* weighted image at the same level demonstrating homogenous uptake of contrast into the external iliac node (dark), which is normal for an uninvolved lymph node. (b) (i) T2* weighted endorectal MRI image superior to the acetabulum pre-iron oxide nanoparticle contrast displaying a normally enhancing external iliac node. (ii) Post-iron oxide nanoparticle contrast T2* weighted image at the same level demonstrating a lack of homogenous uptake of contrast into the external iliac node (bright), which is consistent with malignant nodal involvement. (Courtesy of Dr. Mukesh Harisinghani, Massachusetts General Hospital.)

FURTHER READING

Abrahamsson PA: Neuroendocrine differentiation in prostatic carcinoma. Prostate 1999; 39(2): 135–148.

Albertsen PC, Hanley JA, Gleason DF, Barry MJ: Competing risk analysis of men aged 55 to 74 years at diagnosis managed conservatively for clinically localized prostate cancer. JAMA 1998; 280(11): 975–980.

American Joint Committee on Cancer: AJCC Staging Manual, 6th edn. Springer, New York, NY, 2002; pp. 309–316.

Bostwick DG, Grignon DJ, Hammond ME, et al: Prognostic factors in prostate cancer. College of American Pathologists Consensus Statement 1999. Arch Pathol Lab Med 2000; 124(7): 995–1000.

Carlin BI, Andriole GL: The natural history, skeletal complications, and management of bone metastases in patients with prostate carcinoma. Cancer 2000; 88(12 suppl): 2989–2994.

Catalona WJ, Southwick PC, Slawin KM, et al: Comparison of percent free PSA, PSA density, and age-specific PSA cutoffs for prostate cancer detection and staging. Urology 2000; 56(2): 255–260.

D'Amico AV, Schnall M, Whittington R, et al: Endorectal coil magnetic resonance imaging identifies locally advanced prostate cancer in select patients with clinically localized disease. Urology 1998; 51(3): 449–454.

D'Amico AV, Whittington R, Malkowicz SB, et al: Clinical utility of the percentage of positive prostate biopsies in defining biochemical outcome after radical prostatectomy for patients with clinically localized prostate cancer. J Clin Oncol 2000; 18(6): 1164–1172.

Elgamal AA, Troychak MJ, Murphy GP: ProstaScint scan may enhance identification of prostate cancer recurrences after prostatectomy, radiation, or hormone therapy: analysis of 136 scans of 100 patients. Prostate 1998; 37(4): 261–269.

Epstein JI: Gleason score 2–4 adenocarcinoma of the prostate on needle biopsy: a diagnosis that should not be made. Am J Surg Pathol 2000; 24(4): 477–478.

George DJ, Kantoff PW: Prognostic indicators in hormone refractory prostate cancer. Urol Clin North Am 1999; 26(2): 303–310, viii.

Gleason DF: Histologic grading of prostate cancer: a perspective. Hum Pathol 1992; 23(3): 273–279.

Greenlee RT, Hill-Harmon MB, Murray T, Thun M: Cancer statistics, 2001. CA Cancer J Clin 2001; 51(1): 15–36.

Han M, Walsh PC, Partin AW, Rodriguez R: Ability of the 1992 and 1997 American Joint Committee on Cancer staging systems for prostate cancer to predict progression-free survival after radical prostatectomy for stage T2 disease. J Urol 2000; 164(1): 89–92.

Harisinghani MG, Barentsz J, Hahn PF, et al: Noninvasive detection of clinically occult lymph-node metastases in prostate cancer. N Engl J Med 2003; 348(25): 2491–2499.

Jemal A, Siegel R, Ward E, et al: Cancer statistics, 2006. CA Cancer J Clin 2006; 56: 106–130.

Oh WK, Kantoff PW: Management of hormone refractory prostate cancer: Current standards and future prospects. J Urol 1998; 160(4): 1220–1229.

Oh WK, Hurwitz M, D'Amico AV, Richie JP, Kantoff PW: Prostate cancer. In: Bast R, Kufe D, Pollock R, et al, eds: Cancer Medicine, 5th edn. BC Decker, Hamilton, Ontario, 2000.

Thompson IM, Goodman PJ, Tangen CM, et al: The influence of finasteride on the development of prostate cancer. N Engl J Med 2003; 349(3): 215–224.

Truong LD, Caraway N, Ngo T, et al: The diagnostic and therapeutic roles of fine-needle aspiration. Am J Clin Pathol 2001; 115: 18–31.

Varghese SL, Grossfeld GD: The prostatic gland: malignancies other than adeno-carcinomas. Radiol Clin North Am 2000; 38(1): 179–202.

FIGURE CREDITS

The following book published by Gower Medical Publishing is the source of some figures in the present chapter. The figure numbers given in the listing are those of the figures in the present chapter. The page numbers given in parentheses are those of the original publication.

Weiss MA, Mills SE: Atlas of Genitourinary Tract Disorders. JB Lippincott/Gower Medical Publishing, Philadelphia/New York. 1988: Figs 3.1 (p. 13.15), 3.4 (p. 14.8), 3.5 (p. 14.12), 3.6 (p. 14.13), 3.7 (p. 14.13), 3.8 (p. 14.14), 3.9 (p. 14.11), 3.10 (p. 14.16), 3.11 (p. 14.10), 3.12 (p. 14.18), 3.14 (p. 14.20), 3.15 (p. 14.20), 3.16 (p. 14.21), 3.18 (4.24), 3.22 (p. 14.17).

Prostate cancer therapy

4

Mari Nakabayashi, Robert W. Ross, William K. Oh

INTRODUCTION

Localized prostate cancer diagnoses have increased in recent years with the advent of the serum prostate-specific antigen (PSA) test. In addition, the risk of prostate cancer is strongly tied to increasing age, so it is postulated that an ageing population will lead to continued increases in diagnosis. Local therapies for prostate cancer include surgical and radiation therapeutic approaches, though some patients may require no specific treatment and can be actively monitored. Approximately one-third of patients treated for localized prostate cancer will eventually relapse despite definitive local therapy, demonstrated in many initially as a rising PSA alone.

Prostate cancer cells are regulated at the onset by androgens, in a state of disease typically called "hormone-sensitive" prostate cancer. In this state, the majority of patients with recurrent or metastatic prostate cancer will respond to androgen deprivation therapy (ADT). However, most patients subsequently progress to "androgen-independent" disease, typically manifested by rising PSA after a median duration of 18–24 months in patients with metastases. These androgen-independent cancers remain susceptible to further secondary hormone manipulations for a more limited period of time, but eventually progress to "hormone-refractory" prostate cancer (HRPC) (see Figure 4.1). The median survival of men with HRPC is approximately 1.5 years.[1] In patients with HRPC, chemotherapy is a mainstay of management, though current efforts are looking to enhance available chemotherapies as well as novel targeted treatments and vaccines. This chapter will describe the current overview in the management of prostate cancer.

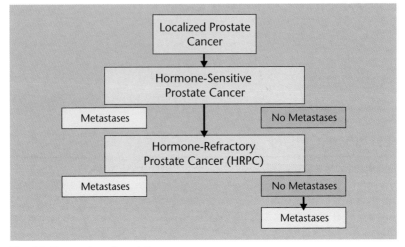

Fig. 4.1 Progression of prostate cancer.

TREATMENT OF LOCALIZED PROSTATE CANCER

Standard treatment options for localized prostate cancer include radical prostatectomy, external beam radiation therapy, brachytherapy (or seed implants) and active surveillance (or "watchful waiting"). Treatment selection is usually made in collaboration with the patient, weighing relevant tumour-related factors such as clinical stage, PSA and Gleason score, as well as patient-related factors such as age, comorbid illness and patient preference.

DEFINITIVE LOCAL THERAPY
Radical prostatectomy
Radical prostatectomy (RP) is generally considered a major option for the definitive treatment of young patients (<70 years old) with localized prostate cancer. Since RP is curative only if the entire tumour is resected, careful preoperative staging is essential. Patients with a low-risk features, including clinical T1 and T2 diseases, PSA ≤10 ng/ml and Gleason score ≤6, have a lower probability of cancer recurrence after RP compared with men with intermediate or high-risk features. Extracapsular extension and seminal vesicle involvement are important negative prognostic features for clinically localized disease, though pathological Gleason score

remains an important predictor of outcome after RP. Nomograms predicting the statistical likelihood of recurrence are available at www.nomograms.org.

The retropubic approach is currently most commonly used due to a lower risk of positive surgical margins, a greater probability of preservation of potency, an opportunity to perform a pelvic lymphadenectomy, and excellent long-term cancer-specific survival rates. Bilateral pelvic lymph node dissection is generally performed prior to RP. However, rates of positive lymph nodes have significantly decreased due to extensive preoperative staging. For patients who have adequate preoperative erectile function, a clinically organ-confined tumour, serum PSA <10 ng/ml, and a digital rectal examination that does not indicate tumour at prostatic apex or posterolateral borders, nerve-sparing RP should be considered, since it is associated with a decreased risk of postoperative erectile dysfunction.

Early complications of RP include haemorrhage, venous thromboembolism and rectal injury, observed in approximately 5–11.5%,[2] 1–1.2%[3] and <0.3%,[4] respectively. Late complications of RP include mild-to-moderate urinary incontinence, reported in 5–13%,[5] and erectile dysfunction. Rates of erectile dysfunction vary widely and usually depend on factors such as the age and baseline sexual function of the patient, as well as how many nerves are spared.

Recently, laparoscopic RP (LRP) has been developed. Advantages of LRP include decreased bladder catheterization, shorter hospital stay, lower margin positivity and decreased intraoperative blood loss.[6,7] Functional advantages such as sexual function and urinary control are difficult to assess because these factors are influenced by the experience of the surgeon, the type of evaluation and the patient's age. The most significant limitation of LRP is that it requires a steep learning curve and advanced laparoscopic skills.

More recently, robot-assisted RP (RARP) procedures have been receiving increased attention because it improves the learning curve compared with conventional LRP. RARP provides 3-dimensional, 10–15-fold magnification visualization, wristed instrumentation, good eye-hand coordination enabled by the robotic system, and a comfortable seated position for the surgeon. It has been suggested that laparoscopic procedures, with or without robotic assistance, are accompanied by less bleeding and pain than conventional RP.[8] Moreover, in non-randomized comparisons, operating times, PSA recurrence and the median time to urinary continence and sexual function appeared to be lowest for RARP. However, the cost for RARP is often significantly more than conventional RP. In addition, since there are no prospective randomized trials comparing either LRP or RARP to conventional surgery, no definitive conclusion regarding cancer control or side effects with these minimally invasive procedures can be made at this time.

External beam radiation therapy

In the last decade, radiation oncologists have refined the technique of external beam radiation therapy (EBRT) with the development of three-dimensional conformal radiotherapy (3D-CRT), using numerous high-energy photon fields and computer software to integrate computed tomography images of the patient's anatomy. This enables the volume receiving the high dose to "conform" more accurately to the shape of the tumour. More recently, intensity-modulated radiotherapy (IMRT) has become available, which allows further refinements of 3D-CRT.[9] IMRT is an advanced form of 3D-CRT that more precisely targets a high dose of radiation to the prostate, while excluding the surrounding normal tissue as much as possible, which may further reduce toxicity.

The volume irradiated includes the prostate and part or all of the seminal vesicles dependent on the calculated risk of their involvement. Treatment is usually conducted 5 days a week, delivering 1.8–2 Gy daily to a total dose of 70–78 Gy. Each treatment session lasts approximately 10–20 minutes. The value of irradiation of the pelvic lymph nodes is controversial, and there is currently no indication to do this in good prognosis localized disease.

Patients with active inflammatory disease of the rectum, previous pelvic radiation, very low bladder capacity, and chronic moderate or severe diarrhoea are contraindicated for EBRT. The common side effects, including urinary symptoms (e.g. dysuria, nocturia), and rectal symptoms (e.g. diarrhoea, proctitis), are usually self-limiting and mild to moderate, but can be severe in a small percentage.[10] In general, with the development of 3D-CRT, side effects on bowel and urinary function have significantly decreased compared with conventional EBRT.[11] Impotence rates following radiation treatment vary from different series but average around 50–60%.

Brachytherapy

Brachytherapy, also known as seed implant therapy, involves placing radioactive sources in the prostate itself. Currently, there are low-dose-rate (LDR) and high-dose-rate (HDR) techniques. The most commonly used energy sources for brachytherapy are iodine-125 and palladium-103 for LDR and iridium-192 for HDR brachytherapy. Because of patient convenience factors, a relatively short recovery time, and the possibility that it may be less likely to induce erectile dysfunction, brachytherapy has become an attractive treatment option for patients with clinically localized disease. A criticism of brachytherapy was lack of long-term data. There are now increasing data of 10- and 15-year patient outcomes suggesting equivalent long-term efficacy compared with surgery or EBRT.[12,13]

Comparison of treatment options

No data from prospective clinical trials are available comparing RP, EBRT and brachytherapy. A large retrospective study performed by D'Amico and colleagues reported 5-year treatment results with RP, EBRT alone or brachytherapy alone.[14] Patients were stratified into low-, intermediate- and high-risk groups according to clinical stage, pretreatment PSA and biopsy Gleason score. For men with low-risk disease, there was no statistically significant difference in the 5-year actuarial risk of PSA failure between the three groups. Patients with good risk disease (clinical T2a or less disease, PSA ≤10 ng/ml, and Gleason grade ≤6) generally have a favourable prognosis with a 5-year biochemical failure-free survival of over 80–90%.[14] Other populations with intermediate- and poor-risk features have significantly worse outcomes, even when treatment is combined with ADT. For intermediate- and high-risk groups, patients that received brachytherapy were at greater risk of PSA failure compared with RP and EBRT. However, such retrospective data, even if controlled for prognostic differences, cannot substitute for a randomized clinical trial comparing these modalities. Unfortunately attempts at randomized trials, including the recent American College of Surgical Oncology (ACOSOG) SPIRIT trial, have failed due to failure to recruit patients.

In general, patients who consider local treatment should base their decision on their cancer risk, age, general health, the treatment side effect profile, available long-term outcome data and availability of a specific treatment in their community. Treatment options not discussed here include cryosurgery, combinations of EBRT and brachytherapy, hormone therapy alone and others. Controversies will continue regarding optimal selection of any of these modalities for specific patient populations.

WATCHFUL WAITING/ACTIVE SURVEILLANCE

A multicentre randomized controlled trial of the Scandinavian Prostate Cancer Group Study has compared RP and "watchful waiting" in patients with clinical stage T1 or T2 disease, PSA <50 ng/ml and negative bone scans.[15] The primary endpoint of this study was prostate cancer-specific survival. During a median 8.2-year follow-up there were significant advantages in the RP group in terms of prostate cancer-specific death (relative risk, RR=0.56) and overall survival (RR=0.74). However, most of the benefit was seen in men under the age of 65 years. While "watchful waiting" may be a reasonable choice for older men with low-risk prostate cancer, especially when their life expectancy is less than 10 years, younger healthy patients should be advised that there is a risk of cancer progression during active surveillance.

MANAGEMENT OF HIGH-RISK LOCALIZED PROSTATE CANCER

High-risk localized prostate cancer is defined as clinical stage T3 disease, PSA ≥20 ng/ml and/or a biopsy Gleason score of 8–10.[14] The optimal treatment strategy for men in this group remains controversial. Standard local therapies including RP or EBRT (combined with ADT) cure only a subset of patients. It has been generally considered that RP alone is less likely to be beneficial in terms of overall survival in men with high-risk disease due to a high likelihood of micrometastases. Short-term neoadjuvant hormonal therapy prior to RP in T3 disease resulted in no improvement in survival in randomized trials.[16] In contrast, studies in Europe and the US have unequivocally demonstrated that neoadjuvant and/or adjuvant ADT in conjunction with EBRT is superior to ERBT alone in terms of overall survival and progression-free survival in patients with high-risk disease (see Figure 4.2).[17,18] EBRT in conjunction with ADT has become a standard treatment option in patients with newly diagnosed high-risk prostate cancer, but research efforts continue for this group as their outcomes remain poor.

SALVAGE EBRT

The goals of salvage RT are to reduce the risk of local recurrence and distant metastases, and modify prostate cancer-specific death. Salvage EBRT after RP is considered in patients with either a delayed rise in PSA or persistently detectable PSA.

A multicentre study of 501 patients treated with EBRT after RP for a rising PSA showed that the 4-year progression-free probability in this cohort was 45%. A persistent elevation in PSA after RP suggests a local recurrence, residual disease and/or metastatic disease. In these cases, RP pathology findings should be reviewed carefully, and metastatic work-up should be considered. Patients with positive margins and other suggestions of persistent locoregional disease should be considered for salvage radiotherapy.

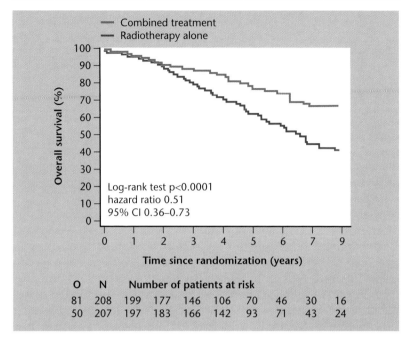

Fig. 4.2 Kaplan-Meier estimate of overall survival. Radiotherapy versus radiotherapy plus hormone therapy. O, Number of deaths; N, number of patients. Reproduced with permission from Bolla M, Collette L, Blank L, et al: Long-term results with immediate androgen suppression and external irradiation in patients with locally advanced prostate cancer (an EORTC study): a phase III randomised trial. Lancet 2002; 360: 103–108.

HORMONE-SENSITIVE PROSTATE CANCER

METASTATIC DISEASE AT PRESENTATION

Metastases from prostate cancer typically involve bone in over 80% of cases. These bone lesions include a mixture of osteoblastic and osteolytic elements, though the clinical presentation is usually dominated by osteoblastic (or sclerotic) metastases detectable on a radionuclide bone scan. Common sites for bone metastases include vertebral bodies, pelvic bones, sternum, ribs and femurs. Lymph nodes are also commonly involved in approximately a third or more patients, generally in the abdomen and pelvis but involvement could be disseminated. Liver and lung metastases are less common, but can occur in up to 10% of patients.

Parenchymal brain metastases are rare, though skull involvement affecting cranial nerves is more common. ADT is the mainstay of treatment for patients presenting with metastatic disease at diagnosis.

ANDROGEN DEPRIVATION THERAPY

It has been over 60 years since Huggins and Hodges published their initial report that prostate cancer is sensitive to androgen deprivation.[19] The goal of ADT is to achieve castrate levels of serum testosterone by either bilateral orchiectomy or medically through the use of luteinizing hormone-releasing hormone (LHRH) analogues. Multicentre randomized trials have demonstrated that these approaches are equally effective.[20]

In the late 1960s, a placebo-controlled study conducted by the Veterans Administration Co-operative Urological Research Group (VAC-URG) suggested that castration is an effective therapeutic modality in palliation of metastatic prostate cancer.[21] In the modern era, the most commonly used method to achieve castration is the use of LHRH analogues such as leuprolide and goserelin. Castrate levels of serum testosterone, generally less than 50 ng/dl, are achieved within 2–3 weeks after the initiation of therapy. Formulation of LHRH analogues now exist in 1-, 3-, 4- and 6-month depot injections, which are required to continuously achieve castrate levels of testosterone. Common side effects of ADT include hot flashes, fatigue, decreased libido, erectile dysfunction, decreased muscle mass, gynaecomastia, weight gain, mood changes, anaemia and osteoporosis. The degree of side effects that affect the patient's quality of life varies among individuals. Over 90% of patients with metastatic disease who undergo ADT for hormone-sensitive prostate cancer achieve a significant decline in PSA as well as a palliative response. The median duration or response in metastatic patients is approximately 18–24 months.

COMBINED ANDROGEN BLOCKADE

For decades, it has been suggested that low levels of adrenal androgens are implicated in the proliferation of prostate cancer cells in men who have undergone testicular androgen ablation.[22] Indeed surgeons in the 1960s reported responses to bilateral adrenalectomy in patients progressing with metastatic disease after bilateral orchiectomy. The concept of combined androgen blockade (CAB) evolved to attempt to achieve maximal blockade of testosterone, by using androgen receptor blockade, adding blockade of adrenal testosterone to LHRH analogue.[23]

The concept that CAB may be superior to ADT alone has been tested in randomized trials. A large randomized trial of 603 men with metastatic hormone-sensitive prostate cancer treated with leuprolide or leuprolide plus flutamide showed that median survival was slightly longer in the CAB arm than the leuprolide alone arm (35.6 vs. 28.3 months, ρ=0.035).[24] Symptomatic improvement was greatest during the first 3 months of CAB, while leuprolide alone often induces a painful flare in the bone, understandable given the brief (<1 month) testosterone flare associated with the use of an agonist in this setting. This influential study seemed to confirm that CAB was superior to LHRH analogue monotherapy. However, in a follow-up randomized controlled trial of 700 men performed by the same cooperative group, the addition of flutamide to bilateral orchiectomy failed to demonstrate any significant advantage over surgical castration alone.[25] Interestingly, PSA suppression rates were statistically higher in the flutamide arm, but this did not translate in this study to a survival benefit. Numerous randomized clinical trials have compared CAB with castration alone in metastatic prostate cancer. A meta-analysis conducted by the Prostate Cancer Trialists's Collaborative Group evaluated the data from over 5,000 men participating in randomized trials of CAB versus castration alone (see Figure 4.3).[26] This meta-analysis did not show a clinically meaningful benefit of CAB over castration alone, with a 10-year survival difference of only 0.7% favouring the CAB arm. Considering the toxicity and expense of the additional antiandrogen therapy, CAB is not considered to be of significant additional benefit compared with ADT monotherapy with LHRH analogue or bilateral orchiectomy. The later addition of an antiandrogen to a patient progressing on primary ADT may be considered, however.

Recently more patients are starting ADT in the setting of non-metastatic disease, for instance in the setting of a rising PSA test after surgery or radiation. In such settings the value of CAB is even more poorly understood. In summary, it is important to consider a month of antiandrogen treatment to suppress the testosterone flare during the initiation of LHRH analogues, but beyond that, its ongoing use as a component of CAB remains of marginal benefit.

ANTIANDROGEN MONOTHERAPY

Non-steroidal antiandrogens block testosterone in target tissues by competitively blocking the androgen receptor (AR). There are three non-steroidal antiandrogens commercially available: bicalutamide, flutamide,

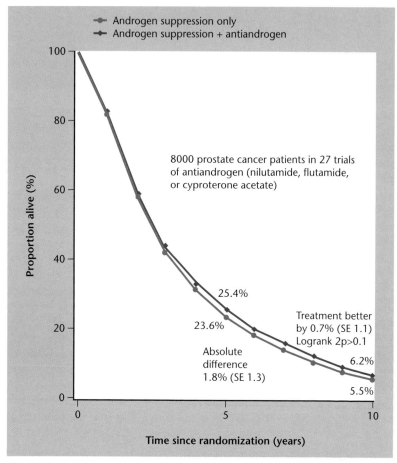

Fig. 4.3 Ten-year survival in the 27 randomized trials of combined androgen blockade (CAB) versus androgen suppression by bilateral orchiectomy and/or the use of luteinizing hormone-releasing hormone (LHRH) analogues. Reproduced with permission from Prostate Cancer Trialists Collaborative Group: Maximum androgen blockade in advanced prostate cancer: an overview of the randomised trials. Lancet 2000; 355: 1491–1498.

and nilutamide. Among these, bicalutamide monotherapy has been extensively evaluated in phase III trials. Several randomized controlled trials have investigated the efficacy of bicalutamide (150 mg qd) and flutamide (250 mg tid) monotherapy compared with castration alone in patients with metastatic prostate cancer.[27,28] In these trials, antiandrogen monotherapy proved inferior to castration in patients with metastatic disease. However, patients treated initially with flutamide notably were not crossed over to ADT, which may have induced a salvage response. In contrast, another more recent multicentre randomized study compared bicalutamide monotherapy (150 mg po daily) versus castration alone in 480 patients with locally advanced disease.[29] Overall survival at 6.3 years of follow-up was similar; however, patients receiving bicalutamide monotherapy showed significantly better quality of life, particularly physical capacity and sexual function.

In addition to its use as monotherapy, antiandrogens have been combined with finasteride to treat hormone-sensitive disease.[30–33] It has been suggested that adding finasteride, a 5-alpha reductase inhibitor, to an antiandrogen may enhance intracellular androgen blockade by lowering dihydrotestosterone levels.[34] A pilot study of high-dose bicalutamide (150 mg/day) and finasteride (5 mg/day) was conducted in 41 men with hormone-sensitive prostate cancer.[33] Finasteride was added to bicalutamide at first PSA nadir. At a median follow-up of 3.9 years, 73% of patients achieved a second PSA nadir with a median decrease of 98.5% from baseline. Median time to treatment failure was 21.3 months. Side effects were mild, but the most common side effect was grade 1 or 2 gynaecomastia and breast tenderness, seen in 61% of patients. This side effect can often be attenuated or prevented by using prophylactic EBRT to the breasts. Sexual function was preserved in 59% and 50% of men at baseline and at second PSA nadir, respectively.

TIMING OF ADT

The Medical Research Council (MRC) conducted a randomized study to ask whether ADT should be started immediately after the diagnosis of advanced prostate cancer or upon signs of clinical progression.[35] Nine hundred and thirty-four patients with locally advanced or metastatic disease were randomized to immediate ADT with either orchiectomy or LHRH analogues (with or without antiandrogen) versus deferred ADT until clinical progression. Development of metastases, skeletal pain and ureteric obstruction requiring transurethral resection of the prostate (TURP) were significantly more common in the deferred arm than the immediate arm. Complications such as spinal cord compression, pathological fractures and extraskeletal metastases were twice as high in the deferred arm than the immediate arm. The prostate cancer-specific death rate was significantly higher in the deferred group than the immediate group (71% versus 62%, respectively, p=0.001). In non-metastatic patients, the difference in survival was 55% for the immediate arm and 52% for the deferred arm. At least part of the modest difference between the groups could be accounted for by the lack of definitive guidelines for when to consider intervention, which was left to individual physicians. Indeed, a significant number of patients in the deferred arm never received any ADT prior to their death. The investigators concluded that earlier hormonal therapy may be preferential, but that deferred ADT may be a treatment option for some older men with non-metastatic disease.

Another randomized trial also suggests that earlier ADT is beneficial, though in a different population with lymph node-positive cancer discovered after completion of RP and pelvic lymphadenectomy.[36] Ninety-eight patients were randomized to receive immediate ADT with bilateral orchiectomy or goserelin 3.6 mg every 28 days versus observation until disease progression (including development of metastases or symptoms). With a median follow-up of 11.9 years, overall survival was longer in the immediate ADT arm than the delayed ADT arm (hazard ratio 1.84, 95%CI 1.01–3.35, p=0.04). Prostate cancer-specific survival and progression-free survival were also better in the immediate ADT arm than the delayed ADT arm (hazard ratio 4.09, 95%CI 1.76–9.49, p=0.0004; 3.42, 95%CI 1.96–5.98, p<0.0001; respectively). The investigators concluded that immediate ADT benefits patients with node-positive disease who have had RP and lymphadenectomy, compared with men who receive delayed ADT. Of note, with more accurate preoperative staging and with the widespread use of PSA as a monitoring test, the clinical applicability of this trial is limited. However, it has been used to suggest that earlier ADT may be useful (namely prior to the development of symptomatic disease). It has not defined a treatment strategy for patients with rising PSA.

A European clinical trial (EORTC 30891) comparing immediate versus deferred ADT with LHRH analogue randomized 985 patients with newly diagnosed T0–4 N0–2 M0 prostate cancer to receive immediate ADT or delayed ADT until clinical progression or occurrence of serious complication.[37] The hazard ratio for overall survival was 1.25 (95%CI 1.05–1.48, p>0.1) favouring immediate ADT. However, there was no significant difference in prostate cancer mortality at a median follow-up of 7.8 years. An additional study is currently ongoing to identify subgroups of patients who will maximally benefit from immediate ADT.

For patients with metastatic disease, immediate ADT is usually warranted, even if the patient is asymptomatic.

RISING PSA STATE

Despite undergoing definitive local therapy, some patients show evidence of rising PSA in the absence of metastatic disease, also known as "biochemical recurrence". It is understood that a continuously rising PSA corresponds to micrometastatic disease. The optimal timing of the institution of ADT in patients with rising PSA is controversial and no randomized prospective data for timing of ADT exist in this patient population. In one natural history series of patients treated with RP and followed with rising PSA without ADT, clinical metastases were not seen for a median of 6–8 years after RP.[38] Though the VACURG study noted earlier suggested that delaying treatment until symptomatic progression of disease did not affect outcome, it is unclear if these data from the 1960s and 1970s in metastatic patients treated with oestrogen therapy can be applied to modern ADT in an asymptomatic, non-metastatic patient.

The US Department of Defense performed a large observational multicentre study evaluating early versus delayed ADT for patients with a rising PSA only after RP.[39] A total of 1,352 men with a rising PSA were divided into either an early ADT group (N=355) for patients who received treatment with a rising PSA and no clinical metastases and a delayed ADT group (N=997) in which patients received ADT only upon developing metastases. They concluded early ADT in patients with a rising PSA was associated with a delay in developing metastases only for patients with a Gleason sum 8–10 or PSA doubling time ≤12 months (hazard ratio 2.12, p=0.01).

To date, an optimal timing of ADT in asymptomatic patients with a rising PSA is unclear. In general, treatment strategies for this population are currently determined based on initial tumour characteristics (e.g. clinical stage, PSA and Gleason score), PSA doubling time, presence of metastatic disease and patient concerns. A prospective randomized trial is needed to answer this question definitively.

MANAGEMENT OF HRPC

SECONDARY HORMONAL THERAPY

Although all patients are initially responsive to ADT, they will eventually progress to androgen-independent prostate cancer (AIPC) manifested usually at first by a rising PSA while on ADT with castrate testosterone levels. Some patients who have received CAB demonstrate a decline in PSA upon withdrawal of the antiandrogen, the so-called antiandrogen withdrawal (AAWD) syndrome (see Figure 4.4). Approximately 20% of patients progressing on ADT demonstrate PSA declines ≥50%, with a

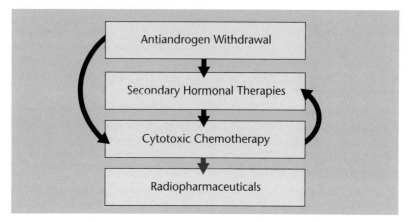

Fig. 4.4 A typical treatment strategy for patients with hormone-refractory prostate cancer.

median duration of 3–5 months.[40] If there is progression after AAWD, prostate cancer may still remain responsive to secondary hormonal manipulation. These include antiandrogens, inhibitors of adrenal androgen synthesis, oestrogens and corticosteroids. None of these agents have been proven to demonstrate a survival benefit. However, these therapies are associated with PSA declines and are usually associated with a mild toxicity profile (see Table 4.1).

SECOND-LINE ANTIANDROGEN THERAPY

Bicalutamide, flutamide and nilutamide are three commercially available non-steroidal antiandrogen drugs. These oral therapies are competitive antagonists of the AR and suppress the effect of circulating androgens, which are primarily derived from adrenal glands in patients on ADT. Antiandrogens have been shown to induce PSA declines ≥50% and symptomatic relief in patients with AIPC.

Phase II studies have shown that 20–25% of patients who were treated with high-dose bicalutamide (150–200 mg daily) experienced a PSA response (defined as a PSA decline ≥50%).[41–43] The most common side effects were hot flashes (23%) and nausea (21%). Flutamide has been shown to have activity as secondary hormonal treatment.[44,45] The toxicity profile is similar to bicalutamide, though gastrointestinal side effects are somewhat more frequent. Both drugs may cause liver toxicity, so monitoring of liver function tests (LFTs) periodically is needed.

Table 4.1 Available secondary hormonal agents and dosing schedules

Treatment	Dosing and schedule	Range of PSA declines ≥50%	References
Antiandrogens			
High-dose bicalutamide	150 or 200 mg po qd	20–25	41–43
Flutamide	250 mg po qd	22	45
Nilutamide	150 mg po qd	19–50	46–49
Adrenal Androgen Inhibitors			
Ketoconazole			
High dose (HDK)	400 mg tid with corticosteroids	28–46	40,93–97
Low dose (LDK)	200 mg tid with or without corticosteroids	27–62.5	50,51
Corticosteroids			
Hydrocortisone	40 mg po qd	16–22	58,98
Prednisone	10 mg po qd	22–34	57,99
Oestrogens			
Transdermal oestrogen patches	0.1 mg/24 hours – 6 patches changed weekly	12.5	56
High-dose conjugated oestrogens	1.25 mg po tid*	25	100
Diethylstilbestrol	1–3 mg po qd*	21–66	52,101–105

* Consider warfarin (1 mg po qd) and/or aspirin
PSA, prostate-specific antigen; HDK, high-dose ketoconazole; LDK, low-dose ketoconazole; po, orally; qd, daily; tid, three times daily

Nilutamide is a third antiandrogen treatment that has been studied in patients with AIPC. Three recent studies have shown PSA responses in 29–50%.[46–48] In one retrospective study, PSA declines ≥50% were observed in 40% of 45 AIPC patients treated with nilutamide 150 mg once daily, with a median time to progression of 4.4 months.[48] However, a prospective phase II study reported a lower response rate in patients with AIPC. In that trial, only 3 of 16 (18%) patients previously treated with bicalutamide had a PSA decline ≥50%.[49] The most common toxicities include delayed adaptation to darkness (unique to this antiandrogen), nausea, LFT abnormalities, and rarely interstitial pneumonitis (<2%). Interestingly, prior antiandrogen use did not preclude the possibility of response to a second antiandrogen, with significant PSA declines reported in several series in as many as 20% to 50% of patients.[43,46,48]

INHIBITORS OF ADRENAL ANDROGEN PRODUCTION

Approximately 10% of total androgen is synthesized in the adrenal glands. Thus, in the castrate state, the adrenal gland is the main source of circulating androgens. Inhibitors of adrenal androgen production include ketoconazole, corticosteroids and aminoglutethimide. Ketoconazole, an imidazole antifungal drug, is the most commonly used agent in this class due to its well-studied activity and generally favourable toxicity profile. A randomized phase III trial (CALGB 9583) investigated the efficacy of high-dose ketoconazole (HDK; 400 mg tid) plus hydrocortisone (30 mg po each morning, 10 mg po each evening) in combination with AAWD compared with AAWD alone in 260 patients with AIPC.[40] Twenty-seven percent of patients showed a PSA response in the HDK arm while 11% had a PSA response in the AAWD-alone arm. An objective response was observed in 20% of patients in the HDK arm with measurable disease, and overall, the median time to progression was 8.6 months. Ketoconazole, however is associated with significant side effects, including fatigue, nausea, vomiting, LFT abnormalities and adrenal insufficiency. Dosage adjustments are not infrequent and occasionally patients are unable to tolerate the drug at all.

Because of these toxicity concerns, low-dose ketoconazole (LDK; 200 mg tid) was studied in a phase II trial and found to have a comparable PSA response in 13 of 28 AIPC patients (46%).[50] Forty-six percent of patients responded, with a median duration of response of approximately 7 months. As expected, toxicity was milder with LDK, including less nausea, fatigue and only one grade 3 toxicity reported (LFT abnormalities). In another retrospective study, 39 of 138 patients (28.3%) treated with LDK had PSA declines ≥50%.[51] Median time to progression or dose escalation on LDK was 3.2 months. Fifty-five patients received subsequent dose escalation to HDK at the time of rising PSA; 12.7% of patients had a subsequent PSA decline ≥50% with dose escalation to HDK. As a result of these findings, physicians can consider starting with LDK with or without concurrent corticosteroids and dose escalate to HDK with steroids in the case of progression or non-response.

OESTROGENS

The pivotal role of oestrogens in the development of prostate cancer has been well supported by data from epidemiological studies and animal experiments. Despite the historical use of oestrogens in the treatment of prostate cancer, little is known about the mechanism of action. Possible mechanism include inhibition of negative feedback on the hypothalamic-pituitary axis resulting in inhibition of pituitary gonadotropin release, direct inhibition of testosterone secretion by the testes and adrenal glands, and possibly a cytotoxic effect on prostate cancer cells.[52] Oestrogen therapies for prostate cancer include diethylstilbestrol (DES), transdermal oestradiol and conjugated oestrogens.

Over 10 contemporary studies of DES in AIPC patients have shown PSA response rates of 21–86%.[52] However, due to an increased risk of serious thromboembolic events and cardiovascular events including death, DES is no longer commonly used in the US as primary ADT, though it is available through compounding pharmacies. A widely available conjugated oestrogens preparation has shown moderate efficacy and modest thromboembolic risk when administered in higher doses with prophylactic low-dose warfarin (1 mg daily). A phase II trial of high-dose conjugated oestrogens (1.25 mg tid) in 28 men with AIPC showed PSA response in 25% of patients.[53] One of 12 patients with measurable disease achieved a partial response. Conjugated oestrogens were well tolerated, though thromboembolism was still reported in 6% of patients, despite use of warfarin.

In contrast to oral oestrogens, some studies have suggested that parenteral oestrogens may not increase the risk of thromboembolic events.[54,55] These findings have been explored in a recent phase II study of transdermal oestrogen performed in 24 men with AIPC. Though the PSA response rate was only 12.5%, there were no thromboembolic events, and levels of factor VII, protein C and protein S were stable during the treatment.[56]

CYTOTOXIC CHEMOTHERAPY

Historically, cytotoxic chemotherapy has been considered to be inactive in prostate cancer. However, results from a series of recent phase II and III clinical trials with newer agents have changed this perception by demonstrating PSA response, objective response, palliative response and, most importantly, survival benefit in favour of chemotherapy treatment. Generally most patients who are candidates for cytotoxic chemotherapy will have progressed through primary ADT and often through one or more secondary hormonal therapies. In this regard, they would be considered truly "hormone refractory". In addition, they often have evidence of metastases, though not always so. At times, such patients may harbour metastases but not be symptomatic. Eventually these patients do progress to increasingly symptomatic prostate cancer and usually have a poor prognosis and quality of life. This section will describe the currently available chemotherapy agents in HRPC.

Mitoxantrone

A Canadian multi-institutional randomized phase III trial first demonstrated the benefit of chemotherapy in patients with HRPC treated in a contemporary era.[57] One hundred and sixty-one men with symptomatic HRPC were randomized to either mitoxantrone (12 mg/m^2) given every 3 weeks plus prednisone (10 mg daily) versus prednisone alone (10 mg daily). The primary endpoint of this study was a palliative response and the secondary endpoints included analgesic use, duration of response and survival. A significant palliative response was observed in patients treated with mitoxantrone plus prednisone compared with the prednisone alone arm (29% vs. 12%, p=0.01). Also patients who received mitoxantrone plus prednisone had a significant longer duration of pain relief compared with patients who received prednisone alone (43 weeks vs. 18 weeks, p<0.0001). There was no survival benefit, however. The regimen was well tolerated except for possible cardiac toxicity in patients who received mitoxantrone, reported in 4%.

Another phase III trial conducted by the Cancer and Leukemia Group B (CALGB) randomized 242 men to either mitoxantrone (14 mg/m^2 every 3 weeks) plus hydrocortisone (40 mg daily) or hydrocortisone alone.[58] The primary endpoint of this study was survival and the secondary endpoints included time to disease progression, time to treatment failure, PSA response and quality of life endpoints. Though there was no significant difference in survival between the two groups (12.3 vs. 12.6 months, p=0.77), patients in the mitoxantrone plus prednisone arm had a longer progression-free survival (3.7 vs. 2.3 months, p=0.025). In a post hoc analysis, a greater number of patients in the mitoxantrone plus hydrocortisone arm had a PSA decline ≥50% (38% vs. 22%, p=0.08), and those patients who achieved a PSA decline ≥50% or ≥80% had a longer survival duration than those that did not (20.5 vs. 10.2 months, p<0.001). Though not statistically significant, there was a trend for improvements in pain control in the mitoxantrone plus hydrocortisone arm. Overall, these two randomized trials suggest that mitoxantrone plus prednisone has clinical benefit in some patients with few available treatment options. Although there was no survival benefit, the US Food and Drug Administration approved mitoxantrone in the management of symptomatic HRPC based on these results.

Taxanes

Taxanes, including paclitaxel and docetaxel, are antimitotic agents that inhibit microtubule depolymerization resulting in cell-cycle arrest. The taxanes have emerged as among the most active chemotherapy regimens

Table 4.2 Taxane-based chemotherapy regimens in hormone refractory prostate cancer (HRPC)

Regimens	Phase	N	PSA decline ≥50% (%)	Measurable response (%)	References
Docetaxel-based					
Docetaxel q3 weeks	II	35	46	28	[106]
Docetaxel q3 weeks + P	III	335	45	12	[68]
Docetaxel q3 weeks + E	III	386	50	17	[67]
Docetaxel q1 week	II	64	64	17	[107]
Docetaxel q1 + P	III	334	48	8	[68]
Docetaxel+ E + Carboplatin	II	40	68	52	[66]
Docetaxel + Vinblastine	II	21	58	60	[108]
Docetaxel + Calcitriol	II	37	81	53	[89]
Docetaxel+ Thalidomide	II	36	53	N/A	[109]
Paclitaxel-based					
Paclitaxel 3q weeks + E	II	34	53	44	[62]
Paclitaxel 1q week + E	II	79	47	N/A	[110]
Paclitaxel q1 week + E+ Carboplatin	II	56	67	45	[66]
Paclitaxel q1 week	II	84	27	N/A	[110]
Paclitaxel q3 weeks	II	23	0	4	[60]

PSA, prostate-specific antigen; P, prednisone; E, estramustine tested to date in prostate cancer (see Table 4.2). In phase II trials, single-agent paclitaxel had shown a PSA response rate of up to 34%.[59–61] However, when paclitaxel is combined with estramustine, studies have shown increased activity by PSA criteria. A phase II trial of paclitaxel (120 mg/m^2 by 96-hour intravenous infusion on days 1 through 4 of each 21-day cycle) and oral estramustine (600 mg/m^2 daily) demonstrated a PSA response rate (PSA decline ≥50%) of 53% and objective response rate of 56%.[62] However, grade 2–4 toxicities including nausea, fluid retention and fatigue were reported in approximately 24–33% of patients. In an attempt to minimize toxicity, later studies with different schedules and less estramustine demonstrated similar PSA and objective response rates, ranging from 42 to 62%, and 15 to 39%, respectively.[59,63–65] Weekly infusions of paclitaxel further decreased toxicity, particularly myelosuppression. A phase II trial of weekly paclitaxel, estramustine and monthly carboplatin showed a PSA response in 67% with a median time to progression of 21 weeks. In patients with measurable response, complete and partial response was seen in 6% and 39% of patients, respectively.[66] Unfortunately, grade 3 and 4 thromboembolic events were seen in 25% of patients, likely due to estramustine.

Docetaxel is a semisynthetic analogue of paclitaxel. In 2004, two landmark phase III trials showed a significant improvement in time to disease progression, palliative response, PSA response and, most importantly, survival with docetaxel-based chemotherapy in patients with HRPC.[67,68] In the Southwest Oncology Group (SWOG 99-16) trial, 770 HRPC men were randomized to receive docetaxel (60 mg/m^2 every 3 weeks) and estramustine (289 mg tid for 5 days every 21 days) or mitoxantrone (12 mg/m^2) plus prednisone (5 mg bid).[67] The PSA response rate was higher in the docetaxel plus estramustine arm compared with the mitoxantrone plus prednisone arm (50% vs. 27%, p<0.001). The median time to progression and measurable response rate were better in the docetaxel arm (6.3 vs. 3.2 months, 17% vs. 11%, respectively). In an intent-to-treat analysis, median overall survival was significantly longer in the docetaxel plus estramustine arm than the mitoxantrone plus prednisone arm (17.5 vs. 15.6 months, p=0.02). Side effects included grade 3 and 5 haematological toxicity, nausea, vomiting and cardiovascular events, all seen more commonly in the docetaxel plus estramustine arm (mostly because of estramustine).

Another phase III trial (TAX-327) randomized 1006 men with HRPC to receive docetaxel in one of two schedules (75 mg/m^2 every 3 weeks or 30 mg/m^2 weekly) versus mitoxantrone (12 mg/m^2 every 3 weeks).[68] All patients received prednisone (10 mg daily). Median survival was significantly longer in the 3-week docetaxel arm compared with the mitoxantrone arm; 18.9 months versus 16.4 months (p=0.009) (see Figure 4.5). The PSA response rate was also higher in docetaxel arms than the mitoxantrone group (45–48% vs. 22%, p<0.001). Palliative response was higher in docetaxel arms than the mitoxantrone arm (31–35% vs. 22%, respectively). Finally, 22–23% of the docetaxel arm had an improvement in quality of life while only 13% of the mitoxantrone arm had a similar response (p<0.01).

Based on the results from these two randomized trials, docetaxel plus prednisone every 3 weeks has become a new standard first-line chemotherapy regimen for HRPC. There are a number of trials using docetaxel as "backbone" to improve the efficacy of chemotherapy.[69] In one such strategy, studies added carboplatin to taxanes for the purpose of additive and/or synergistic effect in HRPC patients.[70] Moreover, clinical trials of new investigational drugs in combination with docetaxel are currently ongoing. A recent study showed, though not prospective, that

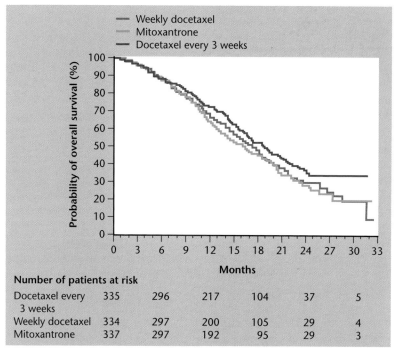

Number of patients at risk

Docetaxel every 3 weeks	335	296	217	104	37	5
Weekly docetaxel	334	297	200	105	29	4
Mitoxantrone	337	297	192	95	29	3

Fig. 4.5 Kaplan-Meier estimates of the probability of overall survival. Mitoxantrone plus prednisone versus weekly docetaxel versus 3-weekly docetaxel. Reproduced with permission from Tannock IF, de Wit R, Berry WR, et al: Docetaxel plus prednisone or mitoxantrone plus prednisone for advanced prostate cancer. N Engl J Med 2004; 351: 1502–1512. © Massachusetts Medical Society.

taxane-based chemotherapy is active when it is given before or after mitoxantrone.[71] This finding suggests that taxanes can and should be used as second-line chemotherapy in HRPC, since they appear to retain their benefit regardless of sequence.

Other antimitotic agents

Epothilone B analogues are a new class of non-taxane antimitotic drugs that have shown activity in taxane-resistant cell lines.[72] A multi-institutional phase II study randomized 92 men with chemotherapy-naïve HRPC to receive ixabepilone, an epothilone B analogue, either with or without estramustine phosphate. The combination and monotherapy arms induced PSA responses in 69% versus 44% and measurable responses in 48% versus 32%, respectively. A prominent side effect of ixabepilone is grade 1 or 2 neuropathy, which occurred in 84% though neuropathy often recovered over time. Data from phase III studies of epothilones B analogues as second-line chemotherapy after taxane failure are awaited.

Vinca alkaloids have modest activity in HRPC. A phase III trial randomized 201 patients to receive either weekly vinblastine (4 mg/m^2) with or without estramustine (600 mg/m^2 daily for 6 weeks).[73] Time to progression was significantly longer in patients who received combination chemotherapy compared with vinblastine alone (3.7 vs. 2.2 months, p<0.0001), though there was no statistical significant difference in survival (11.9 vs. 9.2 months, p=0.08). Vinorelbine and etoposide have also been studied and showed modest antitumour activity when combined with estramustine. Table 4.3 summarizes non-taxane chemotherapy trials.

Timing of chemotherapy

Docetaxel every 3 weeks plus prednisone is approved for the management of HRPC with metastases. Symptomatic disease is not necessary, and indeed many patients who participated in the pivotal phase III trials were asymptomatic. There are no data yet available which suggest that chemotherapy benefits patients in earlier states of disease, including the non-metastatic patient with HRPC, the hormone-naïve rising PSA patient or the high-risk localized disease patient. Ongoing clinical trials are investigating earlier use of chemotherapy in each of these settings, but no definite proof of benefit exists.

Another burgeoning area of need is that of second-line chemotherapy, and in particular, what to do after progression on docetaxel. A large randomized clinical trial is currently investigating the novel platinum drug satraplatin in this group of patients. Other studies are needed to explore new agents.

Table 4.3 Non-taxane chemotherapy in hormone-refractory prostate cancer (HRPC). Selected studies

Regimens	Phase	N	PSA decline ≥50% (%)	Measurable response (%)	References
Mitoxantrone + P	III	384	27	11	[67]
	III	337	32	7	[68]
KAVE	II	46	67	75	[111]
Vinblastine + E	III	95	25.2	20 (PR)	[73]
Vinblastine alone	III	98	3.2	6 (PR)	[73]
E + Etoposide	II	62	39	53	[112]
Vinorelbine	II	49	13	N/A	[113]
	II	47	17	N/A	[68]
Vinorelbine + E	II	25	24	0	[114]
	II	25	38	N/A	[115]

PSA, prostate-specific antigen; P, prednisone; KAVE, doxorubicin + ketoconazole alternating with vinblastine + estramustine; E, estramustine; PR, partial response in measurable disease

BONE-DIRECTED THERAPY

As noted earlier, skeletal complications are a major cause of morbidity in men with prostate cancer. More than 80% of patients with advanced prostate cancer have bone metastases and experience symptoms that include pain, skeletal fractures and spinal cord compression. Together with ADT, which contributes to osteoporosis in men, skeletal comorbidity is a serious problem and significantly affects patients' quality of life. Targeting bone in prostate cancer is an active area of laboratory and clinical research and has led to several therapeutic interventions.

BISPHOSPHONATES

Bisphosphonates are pyrophosphate analogues that inhibit normal and pathological osteoclast-mediated bone resorption. They have recently emerged as a key therapeutic strategy in the management of bone metastases. Several clinical trials have proven that bisphosphonates are effective in reducing skeletal complications in cancer patients. The third-generation bisphosphonate zoledronic acid is more potent than the first-generation bisphosphonate clodronate and the second-generation bisphosphonate pamidronate. In a phase III clinical trial with zoledronic acid, 643 patients with metastatic HRPC were randomized to placebo or 4 mg of zoledronic acid once every 3 weeks. After 24 months of follow-up, the proportion of patients experiencing at least one skeletal complication was significantly lower with 4 mg zoledronic acid over placebo (38% vs. 49%, p=0.028), and the median time to the first skeletal related event was longer in the 4 mg zoledronic acid arm than placebo (16.1 months vs. 10.6 months, p=0.005). Overall, treatment with 4 mg zoledronic acid was associated with a 36% reduction in risk of skeletal complications (p=0.002). Based on this study, zoledronic acid was approved for the management of skeletal metastases in patients with androgen-independent prostate cancer.

The most commonly reported adverse effects include mild-to-moderate fatigue, myalgia and fever. One unique side effect, though rare, is osteonecrosis of the jaw.[74] The optimal frequency and overall duration of zoledronic acid treatment remain questions undergoing continued investigation. Careful monitoring of renal function is required before and during the treatment due to its renal toxicity.

RADIATION THERAPY FOR BONE METASTASES

Radiotherapy has been a mainstay in the palliation of painful bone metastases in patients with HRPC. In addition to pain control, goals of this treatment include elimination or reduction of the use of narcotics and prevent local tumour growth that would cause spinal cord compression or skeletal fractures. Palliative radiotherapy for bone lesions consists of external beam radiation therapy and radiopharmaceuticals.

External beam radiation therapy

Local-field EBRT is particularly effective in the palliation of symptomatic bony lesions. About 50–80% of patients who have bone pain usually experience reduction or relief in pain after the treatment. However, its indication is limited to patients with only a few sites of disease. A 2-week course with 10 treatments given to a total dose of 30 Gy is the standard course of palliative radiotherapy, although there are considerable data demonstrating similar benefit with a single fraction (8 Gy) of radiation,[75] and this schedule is the most commonly used in Europe. Some patients may experience pain flare, which usually lasts 2–3 days at the beginning of the therapy and may be a good predictor of palliative response. Pain relief will often start 1–2 weeks after the initiation of the treatment and should occur within 1–3 months. EBRT is generally well tolerated and acute adverse events are minimal. Patients may feel mild fatigue.

For patients with spinal cord compression from bone metastases to the vertebrae, the management is different depending on the treatment status of prostate cancer. If the patient with cord compression has not received hormonal therapy, immediate ADT and localized field radiation are usually appropriate. If the patient presented with frank cord compression, immediate decompressive surgery followed by radiation therapy should be considered.

Radiopharmaceuticals

For patients with multiple skeletal metastases, radiopharmaceuticals can be considered an alternative treatment option, especially when bone pain is poorly controlled by medication. Radiopharmaceuticals are preferentially incorporated into bone. Several agents, administered intravenously, have demonstrated efficacy in the management of pain associated with bone metastases. Strontium-89 chloride (^{89}Sr), samarium-153 lexidronam (^{153}Sm), and sodium phosphorus-32 (^{32}P) are available radiopharmaceuticals. Strontium-89 chloride is most commonly used in HRPC. Phosphorus-32 is rarely used because of excessive myelosuppression.

Few published data are available on the efficacy and toxicity of radiopharmaceuticals in combination with chemotherapy. A randomized phase III trial of 70 HRPC patients treated with strontium-89 with or without low-dose cisplatin demonstrated that the combination arm had a significant improvement in alleviating pain.[76] Therefore, these agents should be used with caution in patients at risk for thrombocytopenia or neutropenia, since the duration of toxicity can be prolonged.

INVESTIGATIONAL DRUGS

Recent advances in our understanding of the pathophysiology and molecular biology of prostate cancer have led to the identification of a number of treatment targets. Novel agents have been developed targeting angiogenesis, cell-signalling pathways, the immune system, differentiation and apoptosis.

ANGIOGENESIS INHIBITORS

Angiogenesis is required for invasive tumour growth and metastasis, and constitutes an important point in the control of cancer progression.

Thalidomide has known antiangiogenic properties and can inhibit vascular endothelial growth factor (VEGF). As a single agent or in combination with docetaxel, thalidomide has been shown to have activity in HRPC.[77,78] Bevacizumab is a monoclonal anti-VEGF antibody and was tested in a multicentre phase II trial (CALGB 90006) in combination with docetaxel and estramustine chemotherapy.[79] In this study, 79 patients with metastatic HRPC received the combinations, with PSA responses seen in at least 65% and measurable partial responses in 53% of patients. A phase III trial comparing docetaxel plus placebo versus docetaxel plus bevacizumab is ongoing through the CALGB.

CELL-SIGNALLING PATHWAY INHIBITORS

Although the underlying mechanism of HRPC is not fully understood, it is apparent that altered AR signalling plays a central role. It has been postulated that ADT and/or antiandrogen therapy induces clonal selection of "androgen-independent" cancer cells from hormone-sensitive tumours.[80] Recent studies suggested the concept that AIPCs have reactivated the AR signalling pathway by a ligand (androgen) -independent manner, possibly through mutation, amplification and modulation of AR coactivators and corepressors.[81–84] New AR and associated protein inhibitors continue to be developed.

Rapamycin and its analogues CCI-779 and RAD001 are inhibitors of the mammalian target of rapamycin (mTOR). mTOR is a signalling molecule that controls protein required for G1 phase cell-cycle progression.[85] A phase I/II study of RAD001 in combination with docetaxel in men with metastatic AIPC is currently ongoing.

Tyrosine kinase inhibitors (TKIs) include gefitinib (ZD1839), a selective EGFR TKI, trastuzumab, anti-HER-2/neu antibody, and imatinib mesylate (STI 571), an inhibitor of multiple tyrosine kinases including BCR-ABL, c-KIT and platelet-derived growth factor receptor. A double-blind, placebo-controlled randomized phase II trial of gefitinib compared PSA doubling time between the gefitinib and placebo arms (N=58). PSA doubling time was slightly longer in the gefitinib arm compared with the placebo (5.0 months vs. 3.9 months, p=0.25), but no difference was seen in time to progression, and overall survival. A multicentre randomized phase III trial of weekly docetaxel with or without imatinib mesylate was recently completed in patients with metastatic AIPC.[86] Preliminary results suggest that imatinib does not modulate docetaxel activity and more grade 3 adverse events were seen in the imatinib arm compared with placebo.

VACCINES

The goal of immunotherapy is to induce a tumour-specific immune response in the host. Either T-cell mediated or antibody-mediated immune responses may be necessary. Possible target antigens include PSA, prostatic acid phosphatase (PAP) and prostate-specific membrane antigen. Sipuleucel-T (APC8015) is an immunotherapy product containing autologous dendritic cells loaded with a recombinant fusion protein consisting of PAP and granulocyte macrophage colony stimulating factor. It is designed to stimulate T-cell immunity. In a placebo-controlled phase III trial of sipuleucel-T, 127 asymptomatic metastatic HRPC men were randomized to receive either vaccine or placebo.[87] Survival was significantly longer in patients who received sipuleuce-1 than placebo group (25.9 vs. 21.4 weeks, p=0.01). Though not statistically significant, time to progression was slightly longer in the sipuleuce-1 arm compared with placebo arm (11.7 vs. 10.0 weeks, p=0.05). This study is being repeated as a definitive phase III trial.

DIFFERENTIATION AGENTS

Preclinical studies showed that calcitriol, an active metabolite of $1,25$-$(OH)_2$-vitamin D, can induce cell-cycle arrest and cellular differentiation resulting in decreased cancer growth and metastases.[88] A phase II trial of weekly docetaxel plus weekly high-dose "pulse" calcitriol has evaluated the additive effect of calcitriol in 37 men with metastatic AIPC.[89] A PSA decline $\geq 50\%$ was seen in 81% of patients, and 53% of patients with measurable disease had a partial response. The regimen was well tolerated with a toxicity profile similar to single-agent docetaxel. Based on the results from this study, a double-blind, placebo-controlled randomized phase II trial of docetaxel plus DN-101 (a high-dose calcitriol formulation) was performed and results in 250 patients suggested that there might be less toxicity and improved survival with DN-101 given together with docetaxel. This study is being repeated with a survival endpoint.

APOPTOSIS INDUCERS

In vitro studies suggest that the *bcl-2* gene and *bcl-2* protein expression were elevated in HRPC cells compared with hormone-sensitive prostate cancer cells.[90,91] The Bcl-2 antisense oligonucleotide (G3139) oblimersen sodium is designed to target this antiapoptotic gene in order to induce apoptosis in cancer cells. A phase II study of oblimersen sodium in combination with docetaxel in 28 HRPC men showed a PSA response rate of

52% (14 of 27 patients) and an objective response rate of 33% (4 of 12 patients).[92] However, considering the activity of docetaxel, the true added benefit of oblimersen is not conclusive without a randomized trial.

CONCLUSIONS

With an improvement of early detection by PSA screening and of therapeutic options, prostate cancer was only the third leading cause of cancer death in men in 2006, despite being the most commonly diagnosed. Due to the extraordinary heterogeneity of this disease and its complex clinical presentations, appropriate combination and/or sequential therapy is often necessary for better outcome. Accelerated research efforts for new insights into prostate cancer biology and immunology are needed to develop new treatment strategies, ultimately for the improved survival, in patients with prostate cancer.

REFERENCES

1. Smaletz O, Scher HI, Small EJ, et al: Nomogram for overall survival of patients with progressive metastatic prostate cancer after castration. J Clin Oncol 2002; 20: 3972–3982.
2. Koch MO, Smith JA, Jr: Blood loss during radical retropubic prostatectomy: is preoperative autologous blood donation indicated? J Urol 1996; 156: 1077–1079; discussion 1079–1080.
3. Cisek LJ, Walsh PC: Thromboembolic complications following radical retropubic prostatectomy. Influence of external sequential pneumatic compression devices. Urology 1993; 42: 406–408.
4. McLaren RH, Barrett DM, Zincke H: Rectal injury occurring at radical retropubic prostatectomy for prostate cancer: etiology and treatment. Urology 1993; 42: 401–405.
5. Haab F, Yamaguchi R, Leach GE: Postprostatectomy incontinence. Urol Clin North Am 1996; 23: 447–457.
6. Gettman MT, Hoznek A, Salomon L, et al: Laparoscopic radical prostatectomy: description of the extraperitoneal approach using the da Vinci robotic system. J Urol 2003; 170: 416–419.
7. Roumeguere T, Bollens R, Vanden Bossche M, et al: Radical prostatectomy: a prospective comparison of oncological and functional results between open and laparoscopic approaches. World J Urol 2003; 20: 360–366.
8. Menon M, Shrivastava A, Tewari A: Laparoscopic radical prostatectomy: Conventional and robotic. Urology 2005; 66: 101–104.
9. Ling CC, Burman C, Chui CS, et al: Conformal radiation treatment of prostate cancer using inversely-planned intensity-modulated photon beams produced with dynamic multileaf collimation. Int J Radiat Oncol Biol Phys 1996; 35: 721–730.

10. Perez CA, Michalski JM, Purdy JA, et al: Three-dimensional conformal therapy or standard irradiation in localized carcinoma of prostate: preliminary results of a nonrandomized comparison. Int J Radiat Oncol Biol Phys 2000; 47: 629–637.

11. Hanlon AL, Watkins Bruner D, Peter R, et al: Quality of life study in prostate cancer patients treated with three-dimensional conformal radiation therapy: comparing late bowel and bladder quality of life symptoms to that of the normal population. Int J Radiat Oncol Biol Phys 2001; 49: 51–59.

12. D'Amico AV, Coleman CN: Role of interstitial radiotherapy in the management of clinically organ-confined prostate cancer: the jury is still out. J Clin Oncol 1996; 14: 304–315.

13. Grimm PD, Blasko JC, Sylvester JE, Meier RM, Cavanagh W: 10-year biochemical (prostate-specific antigen) control of prostate cancer with (125)I brachytherapy. Int J Radiat Oncol Biol Phys 2001; 51(1): 31–40.

14. D'Amico AV, Whittington R, Malkowicz SB, et al: Biochemical outcome after radical prostatectomy, external beam radiation therapy, or interstitial radiation therapy for clinically localized prostate cancer. JAMA 1998; 280: 969–974.

15. Bill-Axelson A, Holmberg L, Ruutu M, et al: Radical prostatectomy versus watchful waiting in early prostate cancer. N Engl J Med 2005; 352: 1977–1984.

16. Aus G, Abrahamsson PA, Ahlgren G, et al: Hormonal treatment before radical prostatectomy: a 3-year followup. J Urol 1998; 159: 2013–2016; discussion 2016–2017.

17. Bolla M, Gonzalez D, Warde P, et al: Improved survival in patients with locally advanced prostate cancer treated with radiotherapy and goserelin. N Engl J Med 1997; 337: 295–300.

18. Pilepich MV, Krall JM, al-Sarraf M, et al: Androgen deprivation with radiation therapy compared with radiation therapy alone for locally advanced prostatic carcinoma: a randomized comparative trial of the Radiation Therapy Oncology Group. Urology 1995; 45: 616–623.

19. Huggins C, Hodges CV: Studies in prostate cancer. I. The effect of estrogen and androgen injection on serum phosphatases in metastatic carcinoma of the prostate. Cancer Res 1941; 1: 243.

20. Vogelzang NJ, Chodak GW, Soloway MS, et al: Goserelin versus orchiectomy in the treatment of advanced prostate cancer: final results of a randomized trial. Zoladex Prostate Study Group. Urology 1995; 46: 220–226.

21. The Veterans Administration Co-operative Urological Research Group. Treatment and survival of patients with cancer of the prostate. Surg Gynecol Obstet 1967; 124: 1011–1017.

22. Geller J, Albert J, Vik A: Advantages of total androgen blockade in the treatment of advanced prostate cancer. Semin Oncol 1988; 15: 53–61.

23. Labrie F, Dupont A, Belanger A, et al: New approach in the treatment of prostate cancer: Complete instead of partial withdrawal of androgens. Prostate 1983; 4: 579–594.

24. Crawford ED, Eisenberger MA, McLeod DG, et al: A controlled trial of leuprolide with and without flutamide in prostatic carcinoma. N Engl J Med 1989; 321: 419–424.

25. Eisenberger MA, Blumenstein BA, Crawford ED, et al: Bilateral orchiectomy with or without flutamide for metastatic prostate cancer. N Engl J Med 1998; 339: 1036–1042.

26. Prostate Cancer Trialists' Collaborative Group. Maximum androgen blockade in advanced prostate cancer: an overview of 22 randomised trials with 3283 deaths in 5710 patients. Lancet 1995; 346: 265–269.

27. Boccon-Gibod L, Fournier G, Bottet P, et al: Flutamide versus orchidectomy in the treatment of metastatic prostate carcinoma. Eur Urol 1997; 32: 391–395; discussion 395–396.

28. Tyrrell CJ, Kaisary AV, Iversen P, et al: A randomised comparison of 'Casodex' (bicalutamide) 150 mg monotherapy versus castration in the treatment of metastatic and locally advanced prostate cancer. Eur Urol 1998; 33: 447–456.

29. Iversen P, Tyrrell CJ, Kaisary AV, et al: Bicalutamide monotherapy compared with castration in patients with nonmetastatic locally advanced prostate cancer: 6.3 years of followup. J Urol 2000; 164: 1579–1582.

30. Brufsky A, Fontaine-Rothe P, Berlane K, et al: Finasteride and flutamide as potency-sparing androgen-ablative therapy for advanced adenocarcinoma of the prostate. Urology 1997; 49: 913–920.

31. Fleshner NE, Trachtenberg J: Combination finasteride and flutamide in advanced carcinoma of the prostate: effective therapy with minimal side effects. J Urol 1995; 154: 1642–1645; discussion 1645–1646.

32. Ornstein DK, Rao GS, Johnson B, et al: Combined finasteride and flutamide therapy in men with advanced prostate cancer. Urology 1996; 48: 901–905.

33. Tay MH, Kaufman DS, Regan MM, et al: Finasteride and bicalutamide as primary hormonal therapy in patients with advanced adenocarcinoma of the prostate. Ann Oncol 2004; 15: 974–978.

34. Fleshner NE, Trachtenberg J: Sequential androgen blockade: a biological study in the inhibition of prostatic growth. J Urol 1992; 148: 1928–1931.

35. The Medical Research Council Prostate Cancer Working Party Investigators Group. Immediate versus deferred treatment for advanced prostatic cancer: initial results of the Medical Research Council Trial. Br J Urol 1997; 79: 235–246.

36. Messing EM, Manola J, Yao J, et al: Immediate versus deferred androgen deprivation treatment in patients with node-positive prostate cancer after radical prostatectomy and pelvic lymphadenectomy. Lancet Oncol 2006; 7: 472–479.

37. Studer UE, Whelan P, Albrecht W, et al: Immediate or deferred androgen deprivation for patients with prostate cancer not suitable for local treatment with curative intent: European Organisation for Research and Treatment of Cancer (EORTC) Trial 30891. J Clin Oncol 2006; 24: 1868–1876.

38. Pound CR, Partin AW, Eisenberger MA, et al: Natural history of progression after PSA elevation following radical prostatectomy. JAMA 1999; 281: 1591–1597.

39. Moul JW, Wu H, Sun L, et al: Early versus delayed hormonal therapy for prostate specific antigen only recurrence of prostate cancer after radical prostatectomy. J Urol 2004; 171: 1141–1147.

40. Small EJ, Halabi S, Dawson NA, et al: Antiandrogen withdrawal alone or in combination with ketoconazole in androgen-independent prostate cancer patients: a phase III trial (CALGB 9583). J Clin Oncol 2004; 22: 1025–1033.

41. Joyce R, Fenton MA, Rode P, et al: High dose bicalutamide for androgen independent prostate cancer: effect of prior hormonal therapy. J Urol 1998; 159: 149–153.

42. Kucuk O, Fisher E, Moinpour CM, et al: Phase II trial of bicalutamide in patients with advanced prostate cancer in whom conventional hormonal therapy failed: A Southwest Oncology Group study (SWOG 9235). Urology 2001; 58: 53–58.

43. Scher HI, Liebertz C, Kelly WK, et al: Bicalutamide for advanced prostate cancer: The natural versus treated history of disease. J Clin Oncol 1997; 15: 2928–2938.

44. Labrie F, Dupont A, Giguere M, et al: Benefits of combination therapy with flutamide in patients relapsing after castration. Br J Urol 1988; 61: 341–346.

45. Miyake H, Hara I, Eto H: Clinical outcome of maximum androgen blockade using flutamide as second-line hormonal therapy for hormone-refractory prostate cancer. BJU Int 2005; 96: 791–795.

46. Desai A, Stadler WM, Vogelzang NJ: Nilutamide: possible utility as a second-line hormonal agent. Urology 2001; 58: 1016–1020.

47. Kassouf W, Tanguay S, Aprikian AG: Nilutamide as second line hormone therapy for prostate cancer after androgen ablation fails. J Urol 2003; 169: 1742–1744.

48. Nakabayashi M, Regan MM, Lifsey D, et al: Efficacy of nilutamide as secondary hormonal therapy in androgen-independent prostate cancer. BJU Int 2005; 96: 783–786.

49. Davis NB, Ryan CW, Stadler WM, et al: A phase II study of nilutamide in men with prostate cancer after the failure of flutamide or bicalutamide therapy. BJU Int 2005; 96: 787–790.

50. Harris KA, Weinberg V, Bok RA, et al: Low dose ketoconazole with replacement doses of hydrocortisone in patients with progressive androgen independent prostate cancer. J Urol 2002; 168: 542–545.

51. Nakabayashi M, Xie W, Jackman DM, et al: Response to low-dose ketoconazole and subsequent dose escalation to high-dose ketoconazole in patients with androgen-independent prostate cancer. Cancer 2006; 107: 975–981.

52. Oh WK: The evolving role of estrogen therapy in prostate cancer. Clin Prostate Cancer 2002; 1: 81–89.

53. Oh WK, Manola J, Taplin ME, et al: Phase II study of low dose (LD) and high dose (HD) premarin in androgen independent prostate cancer (AIPC). ASCO 2006 Prostate Cancer Symposium. Abstract, 2006.

54. Hedlund PO, Ala-Opas M, Brekkan E, et al: Parenteral estrogen versus combined androgen deprivation in the treatment of metastatic prostatic cancer — Scandinavian Prostatic Cancer Group (SPCG) Study No. 5. Scand J Urol Nephrol 2002; 36: 405–413.

55. Ockrim JL, Lalani el N, Kakkar AK, et al: Transdermal estradiol therapy for prostate cancer reduces thrombophilic activation and protects against thromboembolism. J Urol 2005; 174: 527–533; discussion 532–523.

56. Bland LB, Garzotto M, DeLoughery TG, et al: Phase II study of transdermal estradiol in androgen-independent prostate carcinoma. Cancer 2005; 103: 717–723.

57. Tannock IF, Osoba D, Stockler MR, et al: Chemotherapy with mitoxantrone plus prednisone or prednisone alone for symptomatic hormone-resistant prostate cancer: a Canadian randomized trial with palliative end points. J Clin Oncol 1996; 14: 1756–1764.

58. Kantoff PW, Halabi S, Conaway M, et al: Hydrocortisone with or without mitoxantrone in men with hormone-refractory prostate cancer: results of the cancer and leukemia group B 9182 study. J Clin Oncol 1999; 17: 2506–2513.

59. Berry W, Gregurich, M, Dakhil S, et al: Phase II randomized trial of weekly paclitaxel with or without estramustine phosphate in patients with symptomatic, hormone-refractory metastatic carcinoma of the prostate. Proc Am Soc Clin Oncol 2001; 20: 175a.

60. Roth BJ, Yeap BY, Wilding G, et al: Taxol in advanced, hormone-refractory carcinoma of the prostate. A phase II trial of the Eastern Cooperative Oncology Group. Cancer 1993; 72: 2457–2460.

61. Trivedi C, Redman B, Flaherty LE, et al: Weekly 1-hour infusion of paclitaxel. Clinical feasibility and efficacy in patients with hormone-refractory prostate carcinoma. Cancer 2000; 89: 431–436.

62. Hudes GR, Nathan F, Khater C, et al: Phase II trial of 96-hour paclitaxel plus oral estramustine phosphate in metastatic hormone-refractory prostate cancer. J Clin Oncol 1997; 15: 3156–3163.

63. Ferrari AC, Chachoua A, Singh H, et al: A Phase I/II study of weekly paclitaxel and 3 days of high dose oral estramustine in patients with hormone-refractory prostate carcinoma. Cancer 2001; 91: 2039–2045.

64. Vaishampayan U, Fontana J, Du W, et al: An active regimen of weekly paclitaxel and estramustine in metastatic androgen-independent prostate cancer. Urology 2002; 60: 1050–1054.

65. Vaughn DJ, Brown AW, Jr. Harker WG, et al: Multicenter Phase II study of estramustine phosphate plus weekly paclitaxel in patients with androgen-independent prostate carcinoma. Cancer 2004; 100: 746–750.

66. Kelly WK, Curley T, Slovin S, et al: Paclitaxel, estramustine phosphate, and carboplatin in patients with advanced prostate cancer. J Clin Oncol 2001; 19: 44–53.

67. Petrylak DP, Tangen CM, Hussain MH, et al: Docetaxel and estramustine compared with mitoxantrone and prednisone for advanced refractory prostate cancer. N Engl J Med 2004; 351: 1513–1520.

68. Tannock IF, de Wit R, Berry WR, et al: Docetaxel plus prednisone or mitoxantrone plus prednisone for advanced prostate cancer. N Engl J Med 2004; 351: 1502–1512.

69. Oh WK, Kantoff PW: Docetaxel (Taxotere)-based chemotherapy for hormone-refractory and locally advanced prostate cancer. Semin Oncol 1999; 26: 49–54.

70. Oh WK, Hagmann E, Manola J, et al: A phase I study of estramustine, weekly docetaxel, and carboplatin chemotherapy in patients with hormone-refractory prostate cancer. Clin Cancer Res 2005; 11: 284–289.

71. Oh WK, Manola J, Babcic V, et al: Response to second-line chemotherapy in patients with hormone refractory prostate cancer receiving two sequences of mitoxantrone and taxanes. Urology 2006; 67: 1235–1240.

72. Lee FY, Borzilleri R, Fairchild CR, et al: BMS-247550: a novel epothilone analog with a mode of action similar to paclitaxel but possessing superior antitumor efficacy. Clin Cancer Res 2001; 7: 1429–1437.

73. Hudes G, Einhorn L, Ross E, et al: Vinblastine versus vinblastine plus oral estramustine phosphate for patients with hormone-refractory prostate cancer: A Hoosier Oncology Group and Fox Chase Network phase III trial. J Clin Oncol 1999; 17: 3160–3166.

74. Migliorati CA, Siegel MA, Elting LS: Bisphosphonate-associated osteonecrosis: a long-term complication of bisphosphonate treatment. Lancet Oncol 2006; 7: 508–514.

75. Wu JS, Wong R, Johnston M, et al: Meta analysis of dose fractionation trials for the palliation of bone metastases. Int J Radiat Oncol Biol Phys 2003; 55: 594–605.

76. Sciuto R, Festa A, Rea S, et al: Effects of low-dose cisplatin on 89Sr therapy for painful bone metastases from prostate cancer: a randomized clinical trial. J Nucl Med 2002; 43: 79–86.

77. Drake MJ, Robson W, Mehta P, et al: An open-label phase II study of low-dose thalidomide in androgen-independent prostate cancer. Br J Cancer 2003; 88: 822–827.

78. Figg WD, Dahut W, Duray P, et al: A randomized phase II trial of thalido-mide, an angiogenesis inhibitor, in patients with androgen-independent prostate cancer. Clin Cancer Res 2001; 7: 1888–1893.

79. Picus J, Halabi S, et al: The use of bavacizumab (B) with docetaxel (D) and estramustine (E) in hormone refractory prostate cancer (HRPC): Initial results of CALGB 90006. Proc Am Soc Clin Oncol 2003; 22: abstract 1578.

80. Craft N, Chhor C, Tran C, et al: Evidence for clonal outgrowth of androgen-independent prostate cancer cells from androgen-dependent tumors through a two-step process. Cancer Res 1999; 59: 5030–5036.

81. Feldman BJ, Feldman D: The development of androgen-independent prostate cancer. Nat Rev Cancer 2001; 1: 34–45.

82. Taplin ME, Bubley GJ, Ko YJ, et al: Selection for androgen receptor muta-tions in prostate cancers treated with androgen antagonist. Cancer Res 1999; 59: 2511–2515.

83. Visakorpi T, Hyytinen E, Koivisto P, et al: In vivo amplification of the androgen receptor gene and progression of human prostate cancer. Nat Genet 1995; 9: 401–406.

84. Chen CD, Welsbie DS, Tran C, et al: Molecular determinants of resistance to antiandrogen therapy. Nat Med 2004; 10: 33–39.

85. Fingar DC, Richardson CJ, Tee AR, et al: mTOR controls cell cycle progres-sion through its cell growth effectors S6K1 and 4E-BP1/eukaryotic transla-tion initiation factor 4E. Mol Cell Biol 2004; 24: 200–216.

86. Mathew P, Thall PF, Johnson MM, et al: Preliminary results of a randomized placebo-controlled double-blind trial of weekly docetaxel combined with imatinib in men with metastatic androgen-independent prostate cancer (AIPC) and bone metastase (BM). J Clin Oncol 2006; 24: abstract 4562.

87. Small EJ, Schellhammer PF, Higano CS, et al: Placebo-controlled phase III trial of immunologic therapy with sipuleucel-T (APC8015) in patients with metastatic, asymptomatic hormone refractory prostate cancer. J Clin Oncol 2006; 24: 3089–3094.

88. Beer TM, Myrthue A: Calcitriol in cancer treatment: from the lab to the clinic. Mol Cancer Ther 2004; 3: 373–381.

89. Beer TM, Eilers KM, Garzotto M, et al: Weekly high-dose calcitriol and doc-etaxel in metastatic androgen-independent prostate cancer. J Clin Oncol 2003; 21: 123–128.

90. McDonnell TJ, Troncoso P, Brisbay SM, et al: Expression of the protoonco-gene bcl-2 in the prostate and its association with emergence of androgen-independent prostate cancer. Cancer Res 1992; 52: 6940–6944.

91. Raffo AJ, Perlman H, Chen MW, et al: Overexpression of bcl-2 protects prostate cancer cells from apoptosis in vitro and confers resistance to andro-gen depletion in vivo. Cancer Res 1995; 55: 4438–4445.

92. Tolcher AW, Chi K, Kuhn J, et al: A phase II, pharmacokinetic, and biological correlative study of oblimersen sodium and docetaxel in patients with hormone-refractory prostate cancer. Clin Cancer Res 2005; 11: 3854–3861.

93. Figg WD, Liu Y, Arlen P, et al: A randomized, phase II trial of ketoconazole plus alendronate versus ketoconazole alone in patients with androgen independent prostate cancer and bone metastases. J Urol 2005; 173: 790–796.

94. Millikan R, Baez L, Banerjee T, et al: Randomized phase 2 trial of ketoconazole and ketoconazole/doxorubicin in androgen independent prostate cancer. Urol Oncol 2001; 6: 111–115.

95. Scholz M, Jennrich R, Strum S, et al: Long-term outcome for men with androgen independent prostate cancer treated with ketoconazole and hydrocortisone. J Urol 2005; 173: 1947–1952.

96. Small EJ, Baron A, Bok R: Simultaneous antiandrogen withdrawal and treatment with ketoconazole and hydrocortisone in patients with advanced prostate carcinoma. Cancer 1997; 80: 1755–1759.

97. Small EJ, Baron AD, Fippin L, et al: Ketoconazole retains activity in advanced prostate cancer patients with progression despite flutamide withdrawal. J Urol 1997; 157: 1204–1207.

98. Small EJ, Meyer M, Marshall ME, et al: Suramin therapy for patients with symptomatic hormone-refractory prostate cancer: results of a randomized phase III trial comparing suramin plus hydrocortisone to placebo plus hydrocortisone. J Clin Oncol 2000; 18: 1440–1450.

99. Sartor O, Weinberger M, Moore A, et al: Effect of prednisone on prostate-specific antigen in patients with hormone-refractory prostate cancer. Urology 1998; 52: 252–256.

100. Pomerantz M, Manola J, Taplin ME, et al: Phase II study of low dose (LD) and high dose (HD) premarin in androgen independent prostate cancer (AIPC). Proc Am Soc Clin Oncol 2006; 24: 4560.

101. Manikandan R, Srirangam SJ, Pearson E, et al: Diethylstilboestrol versus bicalutamide in hormone refractory prostate carcinoma: a prospective randomized trial. Urol Int 2005; 75: 217–221.

102. Oh WK, Kantoff PW, Weinberg V, et al: Prospective, multicenter, randomized phase II trial of the herbal supplement, PC-SPES, and diethylstilbestrol in patients with androgen-independent prostate cancer. J Clin Oncol 2004; 22: 3705–3712.

103. Smith DC, Redman BG, Flaherty LE, et al: A phase II trial of oral diethylstilbesterol as a second-line hormonal agent in advanced prostate cancer. Urology 1998; 52: 257–260.

104. Rosenbaum E, Wygoda M, Gips M, et al: Diethystilbestrol is an active agent in prostatic cancer patients after failure to complete androgen blockade. ASCO 2000; abstract 1372.

105. Shahidi M, Norman A, Gadd J, et al: Prospective review of diethylstilbestrol in advanced prostate cancer no longer responding to androgen suppression. ASCO 2001; abstract 2455.

106. Picus J, Schultz M: Docetaxel (Taxotere) as monotherapy in the treatment of hormone-refractory prostate cancer: preliminary results. Semin Oncol 1999; 26: 14–18.

107. Ferrero JM, Foa C, Thezenas S, et al: A weekly schedule of docetaxel for metastatic hormone-refractory prostate cancer. Oncology 2004; 66: 281–287.

108. Koletsky AJ, Guerra ML, Kronish L: Phase II study of vinorelbine and low-dose docetaxel in chemotherapy-naive patients with hormone-refractory prostate cancer. Cancer J 2003; 9: 286–292.

109. Figg WD, Arlen P, Gulley J, et al: A randomized phase II trial of docetaxel (taxotere) plus thalidomide in androgen-independent prostate cancer. Semin Oncol 2001; 28: 62–66.

110. Berry WR, Hathorn JW, Dakhil SR, et al: Phase II randomized trial of weekly paclitaxel with or without estramustine phosphate in progressive, metastatic, hormone-refractory prostate cancer. Clin Prostate Cancer 2004; 3: 104–111.

111. Ellerhorst JA, Tu SM, Amato RJ, et al: Phase II trial of alternating weekly chemohormonal therapy for patients with androgen-independent prostate cancer. Clin Cancer Res 1997; 3: 2371–2376.

112. Pienta KJ, Redman BG, Bandekar R, et al: A phase II trial of oral estramustine and oral etoposide in hormone refractory prostate cancer. Urology 1997; 50: 401–406; discussion 406–407.

113. Fields-Jones S, Koletsky A, Wilding G, et al: Improvements in clinical benefit with vinorelbine in the treatment of hormone-refractory prostate cancer: a phase II trial. Ann Oncol 1999; 10: 1307–1310.

114. Smith MR, Kaufman D, Oh W, et al: Vinorelbine and estramustine in androgen-independent metastatic prostate cancer: a phase II study. Cancer 2000; 89: 1824–1828.

115. Carles J, Domenech M, Gelabert-Mas A, et al: Phase II study of estramustine and vinorelbine in hormone-refractory prostate carcinoma patients. Acta Oncol 1998; 37: 187–191.

Systemic and mucocutaneous reactions to chemotherapy

5

Joseph P. Eder and Arthur T. Skarin

Cancer chemotherapy is a major component of cancer therapy, along with surgery and radiation. Cancer chemotherapy agents differ from most drugs in that it is intentionally cytotoxic to human cells. This aspect of cancer chemotherapeutic agents produces a narrow therapeutic index (desired vs. undesired effects) for most, but not all, agents in this class. The target of cancer chemotherapeutic agents is the proliferating cancer cell. While many normal tissues are non-proliferating, some are proliferating and toxicity of this class tends to preferentially overlap proliferating tissues – haematopoietic, gastrointestinal mucosa and skin. In addition, each agent often has specific organ toxicity related to its chemical class or unique mechanism of action.

The major groups of cancer chemotherapeutic agents are the direct-acting alkylating agents, the indirect-acting anthracyclines and topoisomerase inhibitors, the antimetabolites, the tubulin-binding agents, hormones, receptor-targeted agents and a class of miscellaneous agents. Despite the disparate nature of this broad class of agents, some generalizations about the effects of chemotherapy are still possible. For more information readers are referred to detailed reports.[1,2]

ACUTE HYPERSENSITIVITY REACTIONS

Acute hypersensitivity can occur with any drug. However, several cancer chemotherapeutic agents are derived from hydrophobic plant chemicals and must be solubilized with agents with a marked propensity for causing acute hypersensitivity reactions, especially histamine-mediated anaphylactic reactions, such as the Cremophor used with paclitaxel. Docetaxel has a lower incidence of this complication.

The incidence of severe hypersensitivity reactions with paclitaxel may be up to 25% without ancillary measures. With antihistamine H1 and H2 blockade and corticosteroids, the incidence falls to 2–3%. Hypersensitivity reactions occur in up to 40% of patients receiving single agent 1-asparaginase but only 20% when administered in combination therapy with glucocorticoids and 6-mercaptopurine, perhaps as a result of immunosuppression. The hypersensitivity usually occurs after several doses and in successive cycles. The reaction may be only urticaria (see Figure 5.1) but may be severe with laryngospasm or, rarely, serum sickness. Fatal reactions occur <1% of the time. Changing the source of enzyme is the appropriate initial step. Two other proteins in

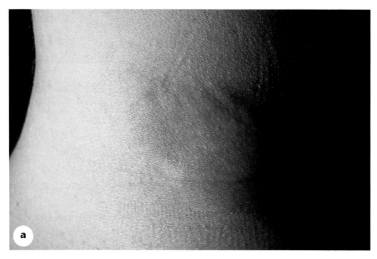

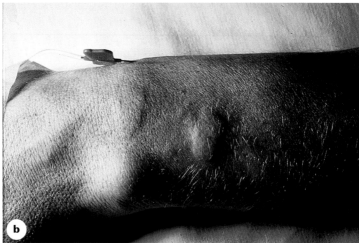

Fig. 5.1 Acute hypersensitivity reactions. Urticaria, with giant localized hives, occurred (**a**) in a 40-year-old man within a few minutes of receiving intravenous 5-fluorouracil and (**b**) in the lower arm of a 50-year-old man after receiving adriamycin. The urticaria was self-limiting in both patients.

clinical use, rituximab and traztuzumab, have a similar incidence of hypersensitivity reactions.

Certain drugs such as etoposide are associated with a greater incidence of reactions but most are not true hypersensitivity reactions. The Tween diluant in the clinical etoposide formulation produces hypotension, rash and back pain. The platinum compounds carboplatin and cisplatin are associated with hypersensitivity reactions, particularly on subsequent cycles – most of these reactions are severe (75%).[3] Hypersensitivity to platinum and related compounds is actually quite frequent, up to 14% in industrial workers, so such reactions in patients receiving these agents parenterally should not be surprising and is often unappreciated in combination chemotherapy regimens, such as with taxanes, and may be equally suppressed by the prophylactic regimens employed.[4] Liposomal encapsulated anthracyclines are associated with an increased incidence of hypersensitivity compared with the parent drugs. Like the reaction to Cremophor EL and radiocontrast agents, the reaction is a "complement activation pseudoallergy".[5] Up to 45% of cancer patients show activation of the classical, alternative or both complement pathways, although the incidence of clinical reactions is about 20%.

Monoclonal antibodies such as trastuzumab, rituximab, bevacizumab, and cetuximab have had enormous impact on cancer therapeutics. Monoclonal antibodies may be chimeric (a murine Fab binding site but human amino acid sequences elsewhere) or fully human. Allergic or hypersensitivity reactions are more frequent with chimeric proteins such as cetuximab (1–5% clinically significant) and are treated with antihistamines and steroids plus slowing of the infusion. L-Asparaginase is a bacterial protein that frequently results in hypersensitivity reactions. These reactions are more frequent with interrupted schedules and with subsequent re-challenge. Changing the source from *Escherichia coli* to *Erwinia* is one accepted strategem if immunosuppression does not work.

ALOPECIA

Many antineoplastic drugs can produce marked hair loss (see Figure 5.2). This includes not only scalp hair but also facial, axillary, pubic and all body hair. The germinating hair follicle has an approximately 24-hour doubling time. Cancer chemotherapy agents preferentially affect actively growing (anagen) hairs. The interruption of mitosis produces a structurally weakened hair prone to fracture easily from minimal trauma such as brushing. Since 80–90% of scalp hairs are in anagen phase, the degree

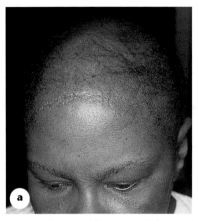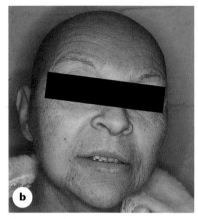

Fig. 5.2 Alopecia. (**a**) Near-total alopecia in a 38-year-old woman receiving cyclophosphamide and adriamycin. Note the loss of eyebrow and eyelid hair. (**b**) Total alopecia developed in this 64-year-old woman due to chemotherapy and cranial irradiation for brain metastases. The duration of alopecia after both treatment modalities may be many months or even permanent in some patients. In this woman, the scalp oedema and erythema are related to an allergic cutaneous reaction from diphenyl hydantoin.

of hair loss can be substantial. Hair loss, while often emotionally difficult for patients, is reversible, although hair may regrow more curly and of a slightly different colour.

STOMATITIS/MUCOSITIS

The oral complications of cancer chemotherapy are many and frequently severe. The disruption of the protective mucosal barrier serves as a portal of entry for pathogens which, especially when combined with chemotherapy-induced neutropenia, predisposes to local infection and systemic sepsis. Once established, these infections may be difficult to eradicate in immunocompromised patients. The most common infectious organisms are *Candida albicans*, herpes simplex virus, β-haemolytic streptococci, staphylococci, opportunistic Gram-negative bacteria and mouth anaerobes.

Several agents of the antimetabolite class of cancer chemotherapeutic agents, especially those that target pyrimidine biosynthesis such as methotrexate, 5-fluorouracil (5-FU) and cytosine arabinoside, and the anthracycline agents, such as doxorubicin and daunorubicin, are particularly toxic to the mucosal epithelium (see Figure 5.3). These agents

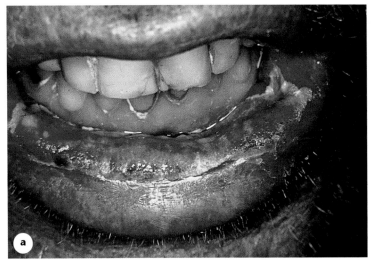

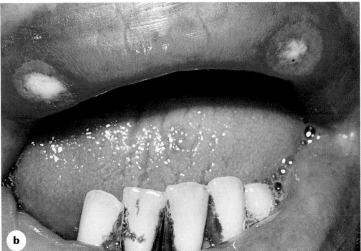

Fig. 5.3 Stomatitis and mucositis. (a) Marked stomatitis in a patient receiving methotrexate. (b) Aphthous stomatitis related to severe granulocytopenia after chemotherapy. The ulcers may be due to herpes simplex or other infection.

have a marked capacity to produce more severe injury in irradiated tissues, even if the radiation is temporally remote. These agents produce marked ulceration and erosion of the mucosa. These lesions occur initially on those mucosal surfaces that abrade the teeth and gums, such as the sides of the tongue, the vermillion border of the lower lip and the

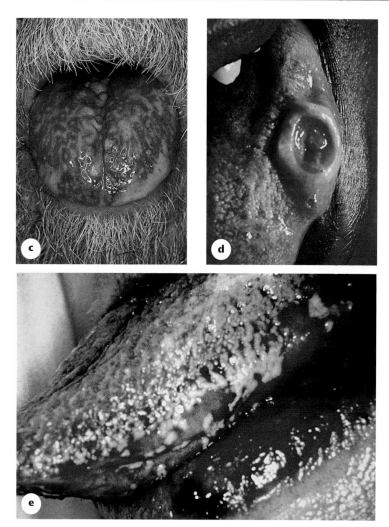

Fig. 5.3 *Continued* (**c**) Mucositis in a patient receiving combination chemotherapy for head and neck cancer. (**d**) Marked ulcer of the tongue in a 32-year-old man receiving induction chemotherapy for acute leukaemia. (**e**) Mucositis of the tongue due to monilia infection (thrush) in a patient receiving corticosteroids for brain metastases.

buccal mucosa. More advanced mucosal injury may occur on the hard and soft palate and the posterior oropharynx. These ulcerations cannot often be distinguished from those caused by infectious organisms. Appropriate tests must be performed to exclude viral, fungal and bacterial causes or superinfection.

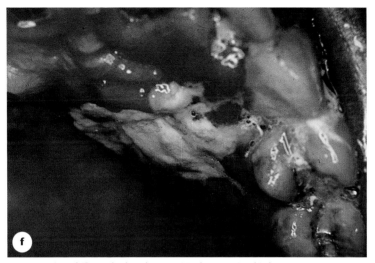

Fig. 5.3 *Continued* (f) Marked oral mucositis due to mixed infection in a patient receiving chemotherapy for acute leukaemia.

In addition to the risk of infection, the resultant pain makes patients unable to maintain adequate nutrition and hydration. This may compromise the capacity to complete a course of chemotherapy and require prolonged administration of parenteral fluids and even parenteral nutrition.

DERMATITIS, SKIN RASHES AND HYPERPIGMENTATION

Superficial manifestations of cancer chemotherapy agents are noted frequently by patients, although they are considered significant much less often by clinicians. The cosmetic changes may be disturbing to patients without requiring discontinuation of therapy.

Of the direct-acting alkylating agents, busulfan has been associated with a wide variety of specific and non-specific cutaneous changes. Diffuse hyperpigmentation has been noted (see Figure 5.4), which resolves with discontinuation of therapy. Systemic mechlorethamine (nitrogen mustard) has no cutaneous toxicity. However, when applied topically for cutaneous T-cell lymphomas, telangiectasias, hyperpigmentation and allergic contact dermatitis may occur. The development of more effective, safer alternative agents has rendered busulfan and mechlorethamine to essentially historical interest only or narrow

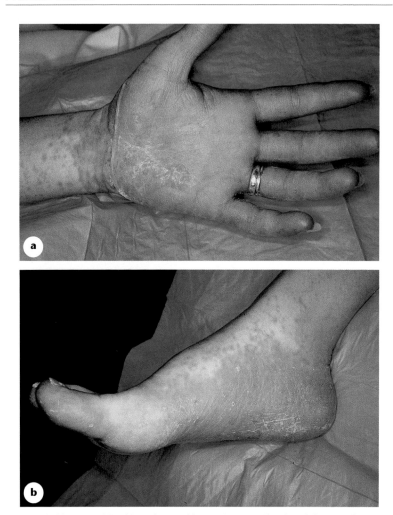

Fig. 5.4 (a,b) Dermatitis, skin rashes and hyperpigmentation: hand–foot syndrome related to 5-fluorouracil chemotherapy in metastatic colon cancer. Note the erythema, oedema, rash and early skin desquamation. Severe pain is associated with this toxic reaction.

indications (busulfan in allogeneic bone marrow transplant for haematological malignancies). Cyclophosphamide, ifosfamide and melphalan produce hyperpigmentation of nails, teeth, gingiva and skin.

The antimetabolites methotrexate and 5-FU are frequently associated with cutaneous reactions. In contrast, the purine antimetabolites

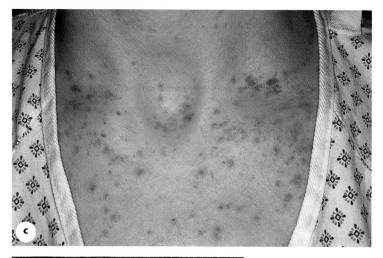

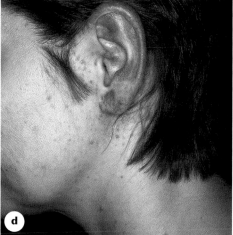

Fig. 5.4 *Continued* (c,d) Skin reaction to Ara-C. Note the erythematous macular rash on the chest and diffuse erythema and oedema of the ears in this 22-year-old woman receiving Ara-C for acute leukaemia.

6-mercaptopurine, 6-thioguanine, cladribine, fludarabine and pentostatin are devoid of cutaneous toxicity. Methotrexate, a folate antagonist, may cause reactivation of ultraviolet burns when given in close proximity to previous sun exposure. This is not prevented by leucovorin, a reduced folate that prevents the myelosuppression and stom-

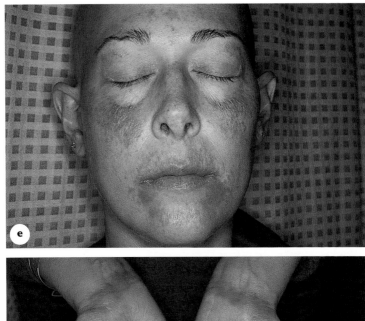

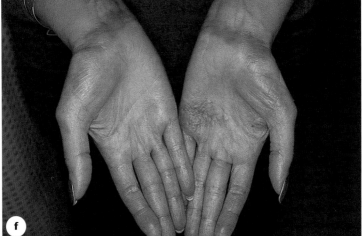

Fig. 5.4 *Continued* (e,f) Skin reaction to docetaxel. Note periorbital and malar flush along with erythema and oedema of the palms in this patient.

atitis of high doses of methotrexate. Methotrexate should be given more than a week after a significant solar burn. It may cause stomatitis and cutaneous ulcerations at high dose, despite the use of leucovorin. Extensive epidermal necrolysis may occur and be fatal. Multiple areas of vesiculation and erosion over pressure areas have been noticed.

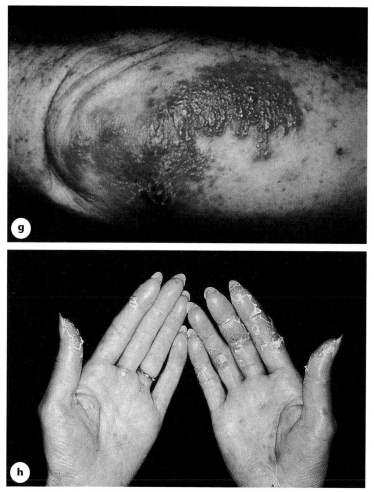

Fig. 5.4 *Continued* (**g,h**) Cutaneous reactions to bleomycin include raised, erythematous and pruritic lesions around pressure points, especially the elbows (**g**), as well as desquamation of skin (**h**).

5-FU is an antimetabolite with steric properties similar to uracil. Like methotrexate, 5-FU produces increased sensitivity to ultraviolet-induced toxic reactions in a large number of patients, over 35% in one study. Enhanced sunburn erythema and increased posterythema hyper-pigmentation characterize these reactions. A hyperpigmentation reaction over the veins in which the drug is administered may occur. This is

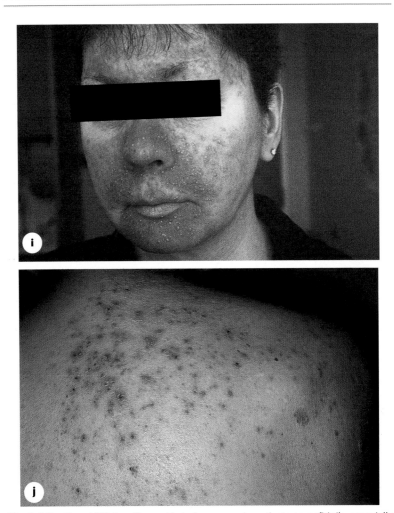

Fig. 5.4 *Continued* (**i,j**) Acneiform skin lesions occur in patients on gefitinib, especially on the face (**i**), chest and back (**j**). These rashes may regress when the drug is temporarily withheld or the dose is lowered. Similar skin reactions occur after actinomycin D and corticosteroids.

probably hyperpigmentation secondary to chemical phlebitis due to chemotherapeutic agents in the superficial venous system. Nail and generalized skin hyperpigmentation have been reported with 5-FU. Occasionally, acute inflammation of existing actinic keratosis is seen in patients receiving 5-FU. This differs from a drug reaction in that it occurs in discrete inflamed regions only in sun-exposed areas, not in a

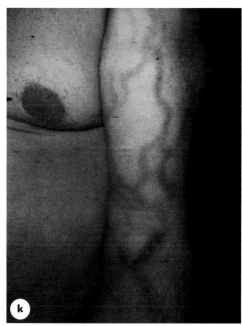

Fig. 5.4 *Continued* (**k**) Hyperpigmentation of the skin along veins occurs after the use of many chemotherapeutic agents, including Navelbine, actinomycin D and 5-fluorouracil infusion, as in this patient. In many cases, the veins become sclerotic due to thrombophlebitis. (**l–n**) Hyperpigmentation of the skin after 5-fluorouracil (**l**), *Continued*

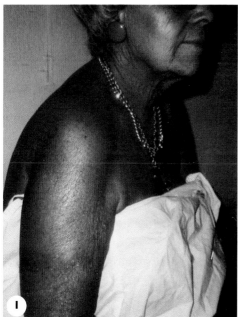

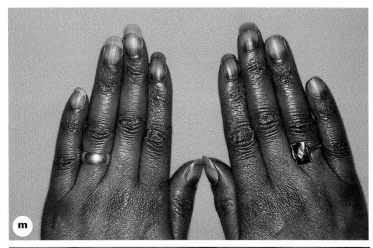

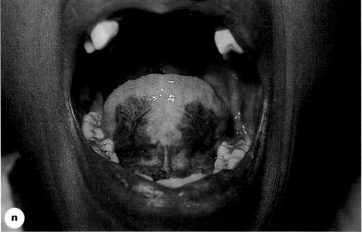

Fig. 5.4 *Continued* Hyperpigmentation of the skin occurs after adriamycin and other drugs (**m**), while increased pigment in the mucous membranes (**n**) and nails (**m**) is mainly related to adriamycin. (Also see Fig. 5.6b).

generalized distribution. The end result is usually the disappearance of the actinic keratosis as a result of an inflammatory infiltration into the atypical epidermis and resultant removal of atypical cells.

When 5-FU is given by intravenous continuous infusion, the most common dose-limiting toxicity is erythromalagia, the so-called hand–foot syndrome (see Figure 5.4). The hands and feet become red, oedematous and often painful. The skin often peels afterwards. The nails become dry and brittle and develop linear cracks. This may occur at doses less than those that produce the hand–foot syndrome. Other drugs that can result in this syndrome include new, targeted therapy drugs, such as sorafenib and sunitinib, which have multiple targets including vascular endothelial growth factor (VEGF) receptor. A similar reaction occurs with 5-FU or 5-FU prodrugs administered orally on a daily schedule. Capecitabine, an oral prodrug that is eventually converted to 5-FU intracellularly, produces erythromalagia as its most common toxicity. Interestingly, oral 5-FU does not produce this syndrome when combined with enyluracil, an irreversible inhibitor of dihydropyrimidine dehydrogenase, the major enzyme in 5-FU catabolism.

High doses of cytosine arabinoside may produce ocular toxicity through an ulcerating keratoconjunctivitis. This may be prevented by the prophylactic administration of steroid eyedrops. Excessive lacrimation may be noted with 5-FU therapy due to lacrimal duct stenosis. This is corrected by surgical dilatation of the duct.

The indirect acting anticancer drugs may produce superficial cutaneous toxicity. The anthracyclines doxorubicin, daunorubicin, epirubicin and idarubicin produce complete alopecia. Radiation recall reactions are frequent, even when the two modalities are separated by years. Skin, nail and mucous membrane hyperpigmentation may be striking; these may be localized or general. Hyperpigmentation of the hands, feet and face may occur in patients of African descent. Liposomal anthracyclines, such as Doxil (doxorubicin) and Daunosome (daunorubicin), may produce a severe erythromayalagia with palmar and plantar erythema and desquamation similar to 5-FU. Actinomycin D produces a characteristic skin eruption in many patients. Beginning 3–5 days after drug administration, patients develop facial erythema followed by papules, pustules and plugged follicles similar to the open comedones of acne. This eruption is benign, self-limited and not a reason to stop therapy. A similar acneiform skin rash occurs in patients taking the new oral epidermal growth factor receptor inhibitors such as gefitinib and erlotinib (see Figure 5.4). In most patients the rash is mild and may regress with continued treatment. When severe, the skin lesions will rapidly regress with discontinuation of the drug. Topical steroids and antibiotics may be indicated.

Bleomycin is actually a mixture of peptides isolated from *Streptomyces verticullus*. Its most common toxic effects involve the lungs and skin because of high concentrations in these organs due to the deficiency of the catabolic enzyme bleomycin hydrolase in these tissues. Cutaneous toxicity occurs in the majority of patients treated with bleomycin doses in excess of 200 mg. Bleomycin causes a morbilliform eruption 30 minutes to 3 hours after administration in approximately 10% of patients (see Figure 5.4). It most likely represents a transient hypersensitivity response (it may be accompanied by fever). Linear or "flagellate" hyperpigmentation may occur on the trunk. This may likewise represent postinflammatory hyperpigmentation. Bleomycin may cause a scleroderma-like eruption of the skin. Infiltrative plaques, nodules and linear bands of the hands have been described. Pathological findings include dermal sclerosis and appendage entrapment similar to that seen in scleroderma. These changes are reversible when the drug is stopped.

Etoposide has relatively few cutaneous manifestations at standard doses (<600 mg/m^2). At higher doses (1800–4200 mg/m^2), a generalized pruritic, erythematous, maculopapular rash occurs in approximately 25% of patients. The most severe toxicity occurs at the highest doses. In these patients, an intense, well-defined palmar erythema develops. Affected areas become oedematous, red and painful. Bullus formation and desquamation follow. The severity of the reaction is related to dose. A short course (3–5 days) of corticosteroids controls the symptoms.

Sorafenib and a related drug, sunitinib malate, are oral multi-targeted receptor tyrosine kinase inhibitors that block signal transduction through the *raf* kinases, vascular endothelial growth factor receptor 2 (VEGFR2) and the platelet-derived growth factor receptors. At the recommended dose there is a 33% incidence of skin rashes or desquamation, 27% incidence of hand–foot syndome and 22% incidence of alopecia (all grades of severity).[6]

Cutaneous rashes are the most common toxicities encountered with gefitinib and erlotinib. The chimeric monoclonal antibodies cetuximab and panitumumab are associated with dermatological toxicity. The severity and extent of the skin changes, including dry skin, desquamation, erythema, nail changes and acneiform eruptions varies from report to report and no consistent grading system for incidence and severity is universally agreed upon. There is neutrophil and macrophage infiltration of the dermis and hair follicles, with thinning of the epidermis and stratum corneum. The incidence and severity is dose-dependent. Certain epidermal growth factor receptor polymorphisms increase the incidence of developing a rash. For erlotinib, cetuximab and panitumumab, several studies support a positive correlation between development of a rash and response, and rash and survival.[7] Management is usually supportive with creams, including 1% clindamycin, 5% benzoyl peroxide and systemic antibiotics when there is evidence of infection, including tetracycline and amoxicillin/clavulinate. These should be used only when necessary.

SKIN ULCERATION AND EXTRAVASATION

Vesicant reactions from extravasated cancer chemotherapeutic agents are one of the most debilitating complications seen with cancer therapy (see Figure 5.5). The anthracyclines, especially doxorubicin, are particularly noted for an intense inflammatory chemical cellulitis caused by

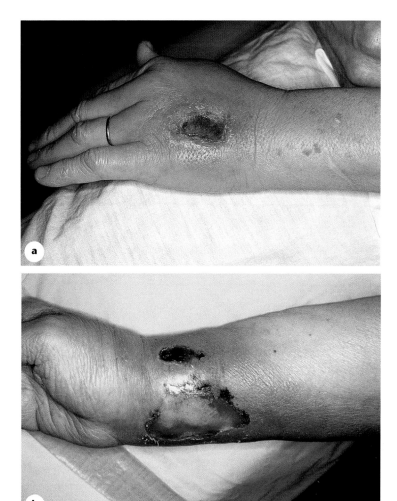

Fig. 5.5 (**a–d**) Extravasation of drugs and skin ulcers occurs with vesicant drugs. Acute changes with adriamycin (**a,b**)

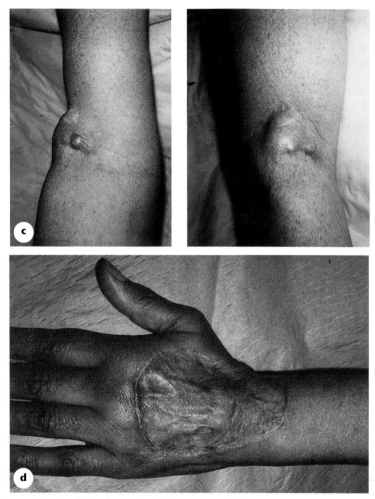

Fig. 5.5 Continued (**c**) Chronic healed scarring with adriamycin, (**d**) mitomycin-C. Other drugs include actinomycin D, vincristine and Navelbine. Immediate medical attention is necessary and sometimes skin grafts are required (see text).

subcutaneous extravasation. This results in ulceration and necrosis of affected tissue. No local measures have proven unequivocally helpful once the accident has occurred. Doxorubicin should be stopped immediately but the intravenous line left in place. Dilution of doxorubicin with sodium bicarbonate and the local installation of steroids prior to catheter withdrawal are standard measures but their efficacy is uncertain. Rest and warm compresses are recommended. If healing does not proceed well, excision of the affected area and surgical grafting are recommended to avoid excess morbidity. Other agents with vesicant properties include the vinca alkaloids (vincristine, vinblastine, vinorelbine) and actinomycin. General recommendations for the administration of vesicant drugs include the use of veins as far away from the hands and joints as possible and that the intravenous line be able to infuse at a rapid rate and have a good blood return. The use of venous access devices is accepted as appropriate in this situation unless contraindicated on specific clinical grounds.

Generalized skin ulceration is an infrequent, albeit dramatic, occurrence. Mucocutaneous ulcerations are frequently noted with bleomycin. These begin as oedema and erythema over pressure points such as the elbows, knees and fingertips and in intertrigenous areas such as the groin and axillae. These areas then proceed to shallow ulcerations. These ulcerations may also occur in the oral cavity. Biopsy shows epidermal degeneration and necrosis with dermal oedema. Total epidermal necrosis can even be found without any dermal changes. This suggests that the epidermal toxicity is the primary event.

NAIL CHANGES

Banding of the nails is the appearance of linear horizontal depressions in the nails that occur as a result of growth interruptions in the nail germinal cell layer by a cytostatic effect from the administration of cancer chemotherapy agents. These occur in other disease settings and are called Beau's lines (see Figure 5.6). The direct-acting alkylating agents cyclophosphamide, ifosfamide and melphalan may also produce hyperpigmentation of nails. The nails may exhibit linear or transverse banding or hyperpigmentation. These changes begin proximally and progress distally and clear, proximally to distally, when the agents are discontinued. Similar effects are seen with the indirect–acting anthracyclines, such as doxorubicin, and bleomycin. The anthracyclines may cause hyperpigmentation of the hyponychia (the soft layer of skin beneath the nail), especially in dark-skinned persons.

Onycholysis is separation of the nail plate from the nail bed (see Figure 5.6). Anthracyclines, anthracenediones and taxanes are the drugs most frequently associated with onycholysis. The combination of these agents is most frequently reported with onycholysis. Most of the reports are associated with docetaxel, either administered weekly or every 3

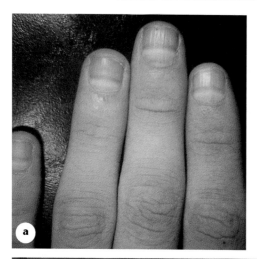

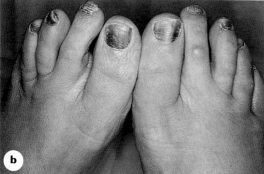

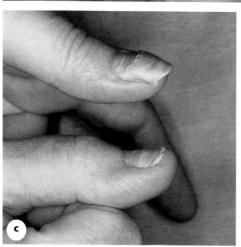

Fig. 5.6 Nail changes are often seen after prolonged chemotherapy. (**a**) Banding of the nails results from growth interruptions in the nail germinal cell layer by the cytostatic effect of chemotherapy. These white bands (called Mee's lines) will grow outward eventually. Beau's lines are transverse grooves across the nail plate due to temporary nail matrix malfunction, seen with chemotherapy or associated with other illnesses (acute coronary or severe febrile episodes). Nail hyperpigmentation occurs occasionally after prolonged use of adriamycin (**b**) especially in people with dark skin. Onycholysis or separation of the nail from its bed is associated with use of adriamycin (**c**), cyclophosphamide and the taxanes.

weeks. These changes occur after hyperpigmentation of the hyponychia, often with hyperkeratosis and splinter haemorrhages. Ultraviolet light may be a facilitating factor. Onycholysis can occur within weeks or months of the initiation of therapy.

RADIATION RECALL

Radiation recall dermatitis is a cutaneous toxicity that develops in patients with prior exposure to therapeutic doses of radiation and subsequent treatment with a cancer chemotherapeutic agent (see Figure 5.7). These reactions occur in the previously irradiated field and not elsewhere. A previous cutaneous reaction at the time of irradiation is not a prerequisite. The onset of symptoms is days to weeks after drug treatment and can occur any time after radiation, even years later. Cutaneous manifestations include erythema with maculopapular eruptions, vesiculation and desquamation. The intensity of the cutaneous response can vary from a mild rash to skin necrosis. Radiation recall reactions in other organs can produce gastrointestinal mucosal inflammation (stomatitis, oesophagitis, enteritis, proctitis), pneumonitis and myocarditis.

An extensive number of anticancer agents have been implicated in radiation recall reactions. The anthracyclines (doxorubicin as an example), bleomycin, dactinomycin, etoposide, the taxanes, vinca alkaloids and antimetabolites (hydroxycarbamide, fluorouracil, methotrexate, gemcitabine) are the most commonly implicated in cutaneous toxicity. In addition, these skin reactions have been seen in association with targeted therapy with drugs such as gefitinib.

Methotrexate and dactinomycin are reported to cause radiation enhancement in the central nervous system (CNS). The antimetabolites doxorubicin, dactinomycin and bleomycin enhance gastrointestinal toxicity from radiation. Cyclophosphamide, taxanes, hydroxycarbamide, doxorubicin, dactinomycin, gemcitabine, cytosine arabinoside and, most importantly, bleomycin exacerbate pulmonary radiation toxicity. Optic toxicity is increased by treatment with fluorouracil and cytosine arabinoside. Radiation lowers the dose of doxorubicin that produces cardiomyopathy.

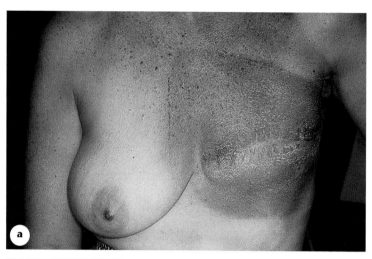

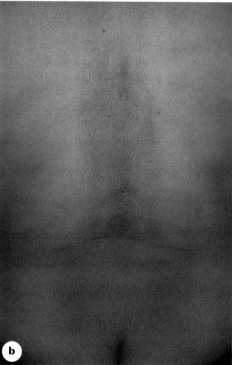

Fig. 5.7 Radiation recall dermatitis may occur in a radiotherapy treatment field after systemic chemotherapy, with development of hyperaemia and then hyperpigmentation in the healing phase (**a**). The patient in (**a**) received adjuvant Alkeran (melphalan) 1 month after postoperative radiation to the chest wall. (**b**) This patient had radiation therapy to the lower spine for bone metastases from breast cancer and developed recall dermatitis 6 months later, when gemcitabine was administered.

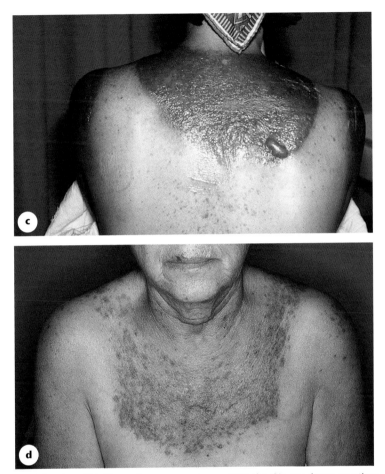

Fig. 5.7 *Continued* **(c)** Chemotherapy can also sensitize the skin to adverse reactions to solar radiation. This young woman developed severe dermatitis in a sun-exposed area while taking methotrexate. **(d)** This patient also developed acute dermatitis in a sun-exposed area while receiving 5-fluorouracil.

ORGAN TOXICITY

CARDIAC AND CARDIOVASCULAR TOXICITY

Cardiotoxicity is a well-recognized consequence of anthracycline use, especially doxorubicin because of its wide spectrum of antineoplastic therapy. This peculiar and potentially lethal problem can be classified as acute or chronic. The acute toxicity is usually asymptomatic arrhythmias, including heart block. Acute myopericarditis occurs at low total doses in an idiosyncratic fashion or at high single doses >110–120 mg/m^2. Fever, pericarditis and congestive heart failure (CHF) are the clinical manifestations. Chronic cardiomyopathy is characterized by progressive myofibrillar damage with each dose, dilatation of sarcoplasmic reticulum, loss of myofibrils and myocardial necrosis/fibrosis. Various syndromes of cardiac toxicity related to antineoplastic agents have been recently reviewed in detail.[8] Imatinib mesylate used commonly in chronic myelogenous leukaemia and gastrointestinal stromal tumours, has been associated with a low incidence of cardiomyopathy syndrome.[9]

A doxorubicin total dose <550 mg/m^2 has a 1–10% occurrence of CHF (daunorubicin 900–1000 mg/m^2), a 40% incidence at 800 mg/m^2 of doxorubicin, and the incidence of CHF approaches 100% at 1 g/m^2. Cardiac function is tested using non-invasive techniques to measure the resting and exercise ejection fraction, including radionuclide ventriculograms and echocardiograms, or invasively by cardiac biopsy. Factors that increase the risk of developing CHF include pre-existing heart disease, hypertension and cardiac radiation therapy. Concomitant dosing with trastuzamab increases the cardiac toxicity of doxorubicin. Cardiac toxicity is a function of *peak* dose level, so continuous infusions or weekly dosing decrease the risk. Desrazoxane, an iron chelator, decreases cardiotoxicity and is approved for use.

Biochemical mechanisms implicated include calcium-mediated damage to the sarcoplasmic reticulum which increases calcium ion (Ca^{++}) release with increased Ca^{++} uptake in mitochondria in preference to ATP. Lipid peroxidations of the sarcoplasmic reticulum, which decrease high Ca^{++} binding sites, and lipid peroxidation due to drug $^\bullet$Fe^{3+} complexes with hydroxyl (OH) radical generation may contribute to cardiotoxicity. The heart has no catalase, and anthracyclines decrease glutathione peroxidase activity, which increases the sensitivity of the myocardium to oxidative damage.

Idarubicin and epirubicin have less cardiotoxicity but are still capable of causing cardiotoxicity. High-dose cyclophosphamide, at doses

>60 mg/kg as used in bone marrow transplantation, can cause a haemor-rhagic cardiomyopathy. Paclitaxel produces clinically insignificant atrial arrhythmias. Agents that can produce arterial smooth muscle spasm may produce ischaemic myocardial infarction in the absence of fixed coronary vascular disease. These agents include 5-FU, vincristine and vinblastine.

Combination chemotherapy in colorectal cancer with bevacizumab has been associated with an incidence (1–3%) of ischaemic cardiac events above that observed with conventional therapy alone. This increase in cardiovascular events, while of low overall incidence, nonetheless represents about a 3-fold increase.[10]

Sunitinib has a 10% incidence of usually reversible cardiomyopathy. Patients can often be treated with lower doses if and when symptoms resolve.[11]

Hypertension has been recognized as a class effect for agents that target VEGFR2. Hypertension is so common that it serves as a pharmacodynamic endpoint in the early development of agents of this class. Hypertension of a moderate degree (grade 2, recurrent or persistent, symptomatic increase of diastolic blood pressure >200 mmHg or to >150/100 mmHg or requiring monotherapy) or severe degree (grade 3, requiring more than one agent or more intensive therapy) occurs in 10–25% of patients receiving bevacizumab, sorafenib or sunitinib. Patients with pre-existing or borderline hypertension are more susceptible. No specific treatment algorithmn has yet been applied to the management of these patients.

PULMONARY TOXICITY

Bleomycin produces pulmonary toxicity, which is the major problem with subacute or chronic interstitial pneumonitis complicated by late-stage fibrosis (see Figure 5.8). The incidence is 3–5% with doses <450 u/m^2, in patients over 70, with emphysema and after high single doses (>25 u/m^2). The incidence rises to 10% at doses >450 mg/m^2, but can occur at cumulative doses <100 mg. Pulmonary injury can occur during high FiO_2 and volume overload during surgery for many years after exposure.

Toxicity results from free radicals produced by an intercalated $Fe(II)$–bleomycin–O_2 complex between DNA strands. Intercalation of drug into the DNA is the first step; then $Fe(II)$ is oxidized and O_2 is reduced to oxygen ($^{\bullet}O_2^-$) or hydroxyl radicals $^{\bullet}OH$. DNA cleavage occurs after the activated bleomycin complex is assembled. Strand breakage absolutely requires O_2, which is converted to O_2^- and $^{\bullet}OH$, and peroxidation products of DNA (and protein) are formed. Free radical scavengers and superoxide dismutase inhibit DNA breakage. Bleomycin is hydrolyzed by

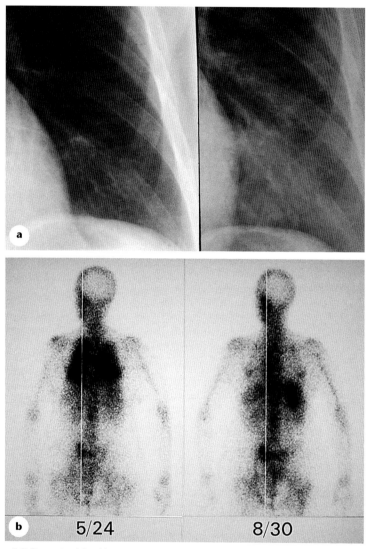

Fig. 5.8 Organ toxicity. Non-mucocutaneous toxicity of chemotherapeutic agents is covered in the text. The lung may be affected by several agents including bleomycin. (a) The earliest radiographic changes are linear infiltrates in the lower lung fields. (b) Gallium-67 uptake is quite striking but is reversible, as this serial study demonstrates.

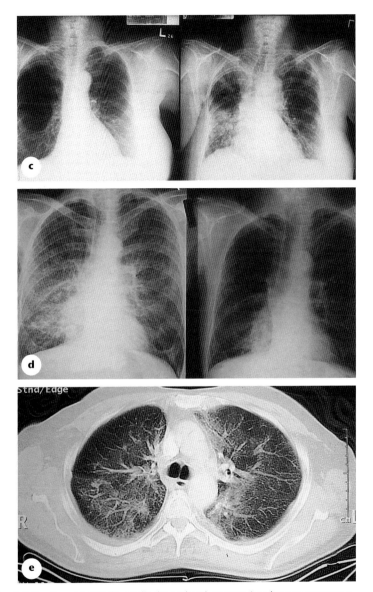

Fig. 5.8 *Continued* (c) While usually dose related, progressive changes may occur resulting in fibrosis and pulmonary insufficiency. Other drugs such as alkylating agents and high-dose methotrexate may result in diffuse infiltrates (d), which were reversible 4 months later. (e) In this patient several courses of gemcitabine resulted in acute dyspnoea and decreased oxygen saturation. Evaluation with lung biopsy and other studies showed no evidence of infection, pulmonary emboli or other diagnosable disease. Use of prednisone led to rapid improvement and regression of the interstitial infiltrates.

bleomycin hydrolase, a cysteine present in normal and malignant cells but decreased in lung and skin.

Busulfan, mitomycin C and carmustine are direct-acting alkylating agents that can cause chronic interstitial pneumonitis and fibrosing alveolitis. This chronic fibrosis produces the clinical picture of progressive, often fatal, restrictive lung disease. The symptoms occur insidiously, often after prolonged therapy. The chronic use of busulfan for the treatment of chronic myelogenous leukaemia is now a historical footnote but carmustine remains the mainstay of treatment for glioblastoma and anaplastic astrocytomas. Cyclophosphamide has been implicated in chronic pulmonary toxicity but rarely as a single agent, more often after radiation.

The antimetabolite methotrexate may produce an acute eosinophilic pneumonitis, which represents an allergic reaction. Cytosine arabinoside and gemcitabine (2',2'-difluoro-2'-deoxycytidine) may also cause an acute pneumonitis, which may be fatal if unrecognized. In these circumstances, withdrawal of the offending agent, supportive care and corticosteroids may prevent a fatal outcome.[12] Some of the reported pulmonary syndromes associated with chemotherapy drugs are noted in Table 5.1.

Table 5.1 Pulmonary syndromes associated with specific cancer chemotherapy drugs

Syndrome	Associated cancer chemotherapy drugs
Pulmonary capillary leak	Interleukin-2, recombinant tumour necrosis factor alpha, cytarabine, mitomycin
Asthma	Interleukin-2, vinca alkaloids plus mitomycin
Bronchiolitis obliterans organizing pneumonia	Bleomycin, cyclophosphamide, methotrexate, mitomycin
Hypersensitivity pneumonitis	Busulfan, bleomycin, etoposide, methotrexate, mitomycin, procarbazine
Interstitial pneumonia/fibrosis	Bleomycin, busulfan, chlorambucil, cyclophosphamide, melphalan, methotrexate, nitrosureas, procarbazine, vinca alkaloids (with mitomycin), gefitinib, erlotinib
Pleural effusion	Bleomycin, busulfan, interleukin-2, methotrexate, mitomycin, procarbazine
Pulmonary vascular injury	Busulfan, nitrosureas

Adapted with permission from Belknap SM, Kuzel TM, Yarnold PR, et al: Clinical features and correlates of gemcitabine-associated lung injury. Cancer 2006; 106: 2051–2057

Both erlotinib and gefitinib, new oral agents targeted at the epidermal growth factor receptor 1, both have a low (<1%) but real incidence of interstitial pneumonitis that resolves if the agent is stopped. The highest incidence is in Asian patients, where 3.5% of patients may develop interstitial disease also referred to as ground glass opacities, which carries a mortalilty of 1.6%.[13]

HEPATOTOXICITY

The liver is a frequent organ for toxicity with cancer chemotherapeutic agents. Centrilobular hepatocyte injury is the frequent histological finding, elevated transaminases the biochemical manifestation. Antimetabolite drugs such as cytosine arabinoside, methotrexate, hydroxycarbamide and 6-Mercaptopurine are all associated with hepatic injury. 6-Mercaptopurine produces a cholestatic picture, with an elevated alkaline phosphatase and bilirubin. L-Asparaginase and carmustine cause hepatotoxicity as well. The injury reverses with discontinuation of the drug. Chronic methotrexate administration, such as in the treatment of autoimmune diseases, is associated with irreversible fibrosis and cirrhosis.

Hepatic vascular injury is another type of injury to the liver associated with cancer chemotherapeutic agents. Hepatic veno-occlusive disease may occur in up to 20% of patients receiving high-dose chemotherapy in conjunction with bone marrow transplantation, with a mortality up to 50%. Jaundice, ascites and hepatomegaly are the full manifestations of veno-occlusive disease but right upper quadrant pain and weight gain occur more frequently. Obliteration of the central hepatic venules and resulting pressure necrosis of the hepatocytes is seen at autopsy. Many regimens and many individual drugs have been implicated. With busulfan, adjustment of the plasma concentration–time profile may reduce the risk. Dacarbazine, a monofunctional alkylating agent, may produce an eosinophilic centrilobular injury with hepatic vein thromboses.

GASTROINTESTINAL TOXICITY

Chemotherapy-induced diarrhoea has been described with several drugs including the fluoropyrimidines (particularly 5-FU), irinotecan, methotrexate and cisplatin. However, it is the major toxicity of regimens containing a fluoropyrimidine and/or irinotecan that can be dose limiting. Both 5-FU and irinotecan cause acute damage to the intestinal mucosa, leading to loss of epithelium. 5-FU causes a mitotic arrest of crypt cells, leading to an increase in the ratio of immature secretory crypt cells to mature villous enterocytes. The increased volume of fluid that leaves the small bowel exceeds the absorptive capacity of the colon, leading to clinically significant diarrhoea.

In patients treated with irinotecan, early-onset diarrhoea, which occurs during or within several hours of drug infusion in 45–50% of patients, is cholinergically mediated. This effect is thought to be due to structural similarity with acetylcholine. In contrast, late irinotecan-associated diarrhoea is not cholinergically mediated. The pathophysiology of late diarrhoea appears to be multifactorial with contributions from dysmotility and secretory factors as well as a direct toxic effect of the drug on the intestinal mucosa.

Irinotecan produces mucosal changes associated with apoptosis, such as epithelial vacuolization, and goblet cell hyperplasia, suggestive of mucin hypersecretion. These changes appear to be related to the accumulation of the active metabolite of irinotecan, SN-38, in the intestinal mucosa. SN-38 is glucuronidated in the liver and is then excreted in the bile. The conjugated metabolite SN-38G does not appear to cause diarrhoea. However, SN-38G can be deconjugated in the intestines by β-glucuronidase present in intestinal bacteria. A direct correlation has been noted between mucosal damage and either low glucuronidation rates or increased intestinal β-glucuronidase activity. Severe toxicity has been described following irinotecan therapy in patients with Gilbert's syndrome, who have defective hepatic glucuronidation. Experimental studies have shown that inhibition of intestinal β-glucuronidase activity with antibiotics protects against mucosal injury and ameliorates the diarrhoea.

Several recently approved receptor tyrosine kinase inhibitors have diarrhoea associated with use, including sorafenib, sunitinib, erlotinib and gefitinib. The frequency varies from 30–40% with less than 5% grade 3 (severe).[14] Also, rare cases of gastrointestinal perforation have been reported using new agents with several mechanisms of action, including inhibitors of tumour vasculature.[15] Hypertension and rare strokes are also side effects that have been reported.

NEUROTOXICITY

Neurotoxicity from cancer chemotherapeutic agents is an increasingly recognized consequence of cancer treatment. The toxicities observed may affect the brain and spinal cord (CNS), peripheral nerves or the supporting neurological tissues such as the meninges. Neurotoxicity from cancer therapeutic drugs must be distinguished from the effects of space-occupying metastatic lesions, toxic metabolic effects from disorders of blood chemistry, adjunctive drugs (such as opiate narcotics) and paraneoplastic syndromes. Toxicity may be acute, subacute or chronic, reversible or irreversible.

The direct-acting alkylating agents ifosfamide and carmustine cause somnolence, confusion and coma at high doses. The toxicity of ifosfamide is secondary to accumulation of a metabolite, chlorethyl aldehyde, in cerebrospinal fluid. Renal dysfunction may cause CNS toxicity at low doses when acidosis results in increased chlorethyl aldehyde levels.

Damage from the antimetabolite methotrexate occurs in three forms and is worse when given intrathecally with radiation. Chemical arachnoiditis, characterized by headache, fever and nuchal rigidity, is the most common and most acute toxicity. This may be due to additives in the diluent (benzoic acid in sterile water). Subacute toxicity is delayed for 2–3 weeks after administration and is characterized by extremity motor paralysis, cranial nerve palsy seizures and coma. This is due to prolonged exposure to high doses of methotrexate. Chronic demyelinating encephalitis produces dementia and spasticity. There is cortical thinning with enlarged ventricles and cerebral calcifications. Types 2 and 3 may be increased after irradiation especially if concomitant systemic therapy with high (or intermediate) doses is used.

Cytosine arabinoside, when given at high doses, produces cerebral and cerebellar dysfunction due to Purkinje cell necrosis and damage. At standard doses, leukoencephalopathy occurs rarely. When given intrathecally, cytosine arabinoside can produce transverse myelitis with resulting paralysis. 5-FU may produce acute cerebellar toxicity due to inhibition of aconitase, an enzyme in the cerebellar Krebs cycle. The purine adenine deaminase inhibitors pentostatin and fludarabine may produce several types of neurotoxicity. Pentostatin produces somnolence and coma at high doses. Fludarabine may cause delayed-onset coma or cortical blindness at high doses, peripheral neuropathy at low doses. Peripheral neuropathy is a frequent toxicity encountered with many cancer chemotherapeutic agents of many classes. Cisplatin and oxaliplatin, the vinca alkaloids and the taxanes all produce peripheral neuropathy in a cumulative dose-dependent manner (see p.73-76 for more on oxaliplatin-related neurotoxicity).

NEPHROTOXICITY

One of the most serious side-effects of chemotherapeutic agents is nephrotoxicity. Any part of the kidney structure (e.g. the glomerulus, the tubules, the interstitium or the renal microvasculature) could be vulnerable to damage. The clinical manifestations of nephrotoxicity can range from an asymptomatic elevation of serum creatinine to acute renal failure requiring dialysis. Intravascular volume depletion secondary to ascites, oedema or external losses, concomitant use of nephrotoxic drugs, urinary tract obstruction secondary to the underlying malignancy, tumour infiltration of the kidney and intrinsic renal disease can potentiate renal dysfunction in the cancer patient.

Platinum compounds are the agents most associated with renal toxicity. Cisplatin is one of the most commonly used and effective chemotherapeutic agents available and also the best studied antineoplastic nephrotoxic drug. It is a potent tubular toxin, particularly in a low chloride environment, such as the interior of cells. Cell death results via apoptosis or necrosis as DNA-damaged cells enter the cell cycle. Approximately 25–35% of patients will develop a mild and partially reversible decline in renal function after the first course of therapy. The incidence and severity of renal failure increase with subsequent courses, eventually becoming in part irreversible. As a result, discontinuing therapy is generally indicated in those patients who develop a progressive rise in plasma creatinine concentration. In addition to this rise, potentially irreversible hypomagnesaemia due to urinary magnesium wasting may occur in over one-half of cases.

There is suggestive evidence that the nephrotoxicity of cisplatin can be diminished by vigorous hydration and perhaps by giving the drug in a hypertonic solution. A high chloride concentration may minimize both the formation of the highly reactive platinum compounds described above and the uptake of cisplatin by the renal tubular cells. Amifostine, an organic thiophosphate, appears to diminish cisplatin-induced toxicity by donating a protective thiol group, an effect that is highly selective for normal, but not malignant, tissue. Discontinuation of platinum therapy once the plasma creatinine concentration begins to rise should prevent progressive renal failure.

Carboplatin has been synthesized as a non-nephrotoxic platinum analogue, but even though it is less nephrotoxic, it is not free of potential for renal injury. Hypomagnesaemia appears to be the most common manifestation of nephrotoxicity. Other, less common renal side-effects include recurrent salt wasting. No significant clinical nephrotoxicity due to oxaliplatin has yet been reported. Limited data have shown no exacerbation of pre-existing mild renal impairment. Studies of oxaliplatin in patients with progressive degrees of renal failure are in progress.

Cyclophosphamide may produce significant side-effects involving the urinary bladder (haemorrhagic cystitis). The primary renal effect of this agent is hyponatraemia, which is due to impairment of the ability of the kidney to excrete water. The mechanism appears to be due to a direct effect of cyclophosphamide on the distal tubule and not to increased levels of antidiuretic hormone. Hyponatraemia usually occurs acutely and resolves upon discontinuation of the drug (approximately 24 hours). It is recommended that isotonic saline be infused prior to cyclophosphamide administration in order to ameliorate this effect.

Ifosfamide nephrotoxicity has a primary renal effect to produce tubular renal toxicity. The damage produced by ifosfamide is concentrated in the proximal renal tubule and a Fanconi syndrome has been observed after therapy. Other clinical syndromes that have been associated with ifosfamide include nephrogenic diabetes insipidus, renal tubular acidosis and rickets. Pre-existing renal disease is an important risk factor for ifosfamide nephrotoxicity.

Carmustine, lomustine and semustine are lipid-soluble nitrosureas, which have been used against brain tumours. The exact mechanism of nephrotoxicity, however, is incompletely understood. High doses of semustine in children and adults have been associated with progressive renal dysfunction to marked renal insufficiency 3–5 years after therapy. The characteristic histological changes include glomerular sclerosis without immune deposits and interstitial fibrosis. The incidence of nephrotoxicity was reported at 26% in patients with malignant melanoma treated with methyl CCNU in the adjuvant setting. Nephrotoxicity has been reported in 65–75% of patients treated with streptozotocin for prolonged periods of time. Proteinuria is often the first sign of renal damage. This is followed by signs of proximal tubular damage, such as phosphaturia, glycosuria, aminoaciduria, uricosuria and bicarbonaturia. Renal toxicity lasts approximately 2–3 weeks after discontinuing the drug.

The most common form of nephrotoxicity associated with mitomycin C is haemolytic uraemic syndrome. It has been reported in patients who were treated with total doses of mitomycin C in excess of 60 mg/m^2. The renal damage caused by this antineoplastic agent appears to be direct endothelial damage. The incidence of this syndrome ranges from 4% to 6% of patients who receive this drug alone or in combination.

Low or standard doses of methotrexate are usually not associated with renal toxicity, unless patients have underlying renal dysfunction. High doses (1–15 g/m^2) are associated with a 47% incidence of renal toxicity, accompanied by methotrexate crystals in the urine. The mechanism for methotrexate-induced nephrotoxicity is explained in part by its limited solubility at an acid pH, which leads to intratubular precipitation. Patients who are volume depleted and excrete an acidic urine are at higher risk for nephrotoxicity. With aggressive hydration and urine alkalinization, the incidence of renal failure with high doses of methotrexate can be decreased. The clinical picture of methotrexate-induced renal failure is that of a non-oliguric renal failure. Preventive measures when using high doses of methotrexate include aggressive intravenous hydration with saline and urine alkalinization with sodium bicarbonate to maintain a urine pH around 7.0. If renal failure develops, methotrexate levels will increase and the risk of systemic toxicity will also be enhanced. In addition to supportive measures, patients should be started on folinic acid rescue, until levels of methotrexate fall below 0.5 uM.

VEGF or VEGFR2-targeted agents produce albuminuria in 10–25% of patients, sometimes to nephrotic range. The exact mechanism has not been elucidated but studies in mice with conditional expression of VEGF in the podocytes confirms a major role for VEGF in endothelial development and maintainence of a fenestrated endothelium.[16] Like hypertension, this appears to be a class effect but the factors associated with occurrence and severity are unknown. If clinically significant, decreasing the dose or discontinuation of drug are the only current approaches.

LATE COMPLICATIONS OF CANCER CHEMOTHERAPY

As cancer therapy has become increasingly effective and more patients live longer, late complications have become apparent separate from the direct toxic effects on organ system function described above. Gonadal dysfunction is one. In males, the primary lesion is depletion of germinal epithelium of seminiferous tubules with marked decrease in testicular volume, oligo- or azoospermia and infertility. There is an increase in follicle-stimulating hormone (FSH) and occasionally in luteinizing hormone (LH). No change is seen in serum testosterone. Alkylating agents (and irradiation) are the most damaging and toxicity is dose related. About 80% of males with Hodgkin's disease treated with MOPP are oligo-azoospermic. About half recover in up to 4 years. Procarbazine is a major offender. Anthracyclines also cause azoospermia in a dose-related fashion. In females, the primary lesion is ovarian fibrosis and follicle destruction. Amenorrhoea ensues, with increase in FSH and LH and a decrease in oestradiol leading to vaginal atrophy and endometrial hypoplasia. Onset and duration are dose and age related. Alkylating agents (and irradiation) again are the worst offenders.

In children, the prepubertal effects may be less profound and reversible in males, though the pubertal effects may be more severe with often irreversible azoospermia, decreased testosterone and increased FSH and LH. Less is known about females, but young girls appear quite resistant to alkylating agents.

No more tragic toxicity is seen with cancer chemotherapeutic agents than the induction of a second, treatment-related cancer in a patient cured of one cancer.[17,18] Of the wide variety of environmental and chemical agents causing cancer, there is one common thread in their mode of action – interaction with DNA. Clinical studies detailing this consequence of therapy have many problems, including the inherent bias of reporting index cases, the retrospective nature of many reports, the lack of reliable information on drug dosage, total amount of drug given and duration of therapy and the underlying incidence of second malignancy. The direct-acting alkylating agents are most often implicated and chronic, low-dose administration is a greater risk factor. Acute non-lymphocytic leukaemia or myelodysplasia is the best described. The indirect-acting topoisomerase II agents produce a specific 11q23 translocation.

Osteonecrosis of the jaw has been seen with increasing frequency during the past few years, related in part to chronic use of intravenous bisphophonates for advanced cancer. The incidence has been estimated at 1–10% of patients receiving these medications.[19] The pathogenesis and optimal management for osteonecrosis of the jaw are poorly understood, with multiple risk factors and various treatments involved.[20]

REFERENCES

1. Weiss RB: Toxicity of chemotherapy – the last decade. Semin Oncol 2006; 33: 1.
2. Crawford J, Cella D, Sonis ST: Managing chemotherapy-related side effects: trends in the use of cytokines and other growth factors. Oncology 2006; 20: Suppl.
3. Zorzou MP, Efstathiou E, Galani E, et al: Carboplatin hypersensitivity reactions. J Chemother 2005; 17(1): 104–110.
4. Cristaaudo A, Sera F, Severino V, et al: Occupational hypersensitivity to metal salts, including platinum, in the secondary industry. Allergy 2005; 60(2): 138–139.
5. Szebeni J: Complement activation-related pseudoallergy: a new class of drug induced acute immune toxicity. Toxicology 2005; 216: 106–121.
6. Escudier B, Szczylik C, Eisen T, et al: Randomized phase III trial of the Raf kinase and VEGFR inhibitor sorafenib (BAY 43-9006) in patients with advanced renal cell carcinoma (RCC). J Clin Oncol 2005; 23(18 Suppl): abstract 4510.
7. Perez-Solar R, Saltz L. Cutaneous adverse effects with HER1/EGFR-targeted agents: is there a silver lining? J Clin Oncol 2005; 23(24): 5235–5246.
8. Floyd JD, Nguyen DT, Lobins RL, et al: Cardiotoxicity of cancer therapy. J Clin Oncol 2005; 23: 7685–7696.

9. Kerkela R, Grazette L, Yacobi R, et al: Cardiotoxicity of the cancer therapeutic agent imatinib mesylate. Nat Med 2006; 12(8): 908–916.

10. Hurwitz H: Integrating the anti-VEGF – A humanized monoclonal antibody bevacizumab with chemotherapy in advanced colorectal cancer. Clin Colorectal Cancer 2004; 4 Suppl 2: S62–S68.

11. Motzer RJ, Hutson TE, Tomczak P, et al: Phase III randomized trial of sunitinib malate (SU11248) versus interferon alfa as first line systemic therapy for patients with metastatic renal cell carcinoma. J Clin Oncol 2006; 24 (18 Suppl): 930s abstract LBA3.

12. Belknap SM, Kuzel TM, Yarnold PR, et al: Clinical features and correlates of gemcitabine-associated lung injury. Cancer 2006; 106: 2051–2057.

13. Ando M, Okamoto I, Yamamoto N, et al: Predictive factors for interstitial lung disease, antitumor response, and survival in non-small-cell lung cancer patients treated with gefitinib. J Clin Oncol 2006; 24: 2549–2556.

14. Niho S, Kubota K, Goto K, et al: First-line single agent treatment with gefitinib in patients with advanced non-small cell lung cancer: a phase II study. J Clin Oncol 2006; 24(1): 64–69.

15. Ratain MJ, Eisen T, Stadler WM, et al: Phase II placebo-controlled randomized discontinuation trial of sorafenib in patients with metastatic renal cell carcinoma. J Clin Oncol 2006; 24: 2505–2512.

16. Erimina V, Quaggin SE: The role of VEGF-A in glomerular development and function. Curr Opin Nephrol Hypertens 2004; 13: 9–15.

17. Bhatia S, Landier W: Evaluating survivors of pediatric cancer. Cancer J 2005; 11: 340–354.

18. Hudson MM, Mertens AC, Yasui Y, et al: Health status in adults treated for childhood cancer: a report from the childhood survivor study. Am J Oncol Rev 2004; 3: 165–170.

19. Badros A, Weikel D, Salama A, et al: Osteonecrosis of the jaw in multiple myeloma patients: clinical features and risk factors. J Clin Oncol 2006; 24: 945–952.

20. Ruggiero S, Gralow J, Marx RE, et al. Practical guidelines for the prevention, diagnosis and treatment of osteonecrosis of the jaw in patients with cancer. J Oncol Pract 2006; 2: 7–14.

FURTHER READING

Adrian RM, Hood, AF, Skarin AT. Mucocutaneous reactions to antineoplastic agents. CA Cancer J Clin 1980; 30: 143–157.

Attar EC, Ervin T, Janicek M, Deykin A, Godleski J: Acute interstitial pneumonitis related to gemcitabine. J Clin Oncol 2000; 18: 697–698.

Burstein H: Radiation recall dermatitis from gemcitabine. J Clin Oncol 2000; 18: 693–694.

Chabner BA, Longo DL: Cancer Chemotherapy and Biotherapy, 2nd edn. Lippincott–Raven, Philadelphia, 1996.

Darnell J, Lodish H, Baltimore D: Molecular Cell Biology, 3rd edn. W.H. Freeman, New York, 1995.

DeVita VT, Jr, Hellman S, Rosenberg SA: Cancer: Principles and Practice of Oncology, 4th edn. Lippincott, Philadelphia, 1993.

Eder JP: Neoplasms. In: Page CP, Curtis MJ, Sutter MC, Walker MJA, Hoffman BB, eds: Integrated Pharmacology. Mosby–Times Mirror International, London, 1997: 501–522.

Hussain S, Anderson DN, Salvatti ME, et al: Onycholysis as a complication of systemic chemotherapy. Cancer 2000; 88: 2367–2371.

Perry MD: The Chemotherapy Source Book. Williams and Wilkins, Baltimore, 1992.

Skeel RT: Handbook of Cancer Chemotherapy. Little, Brown, Boston, 1991.

Sonis ST, Fey EG: Oral complications of cancer therapy. Oncology 2002; 16: 680–691.

Index